Table of contents

Introduction 7

Part 1 : Myths and popular beliefs 8

1. The Butt Wink is dangerous for your back. Avoid the squat or else you will injure yourself! 9

2. I want to tone my body but I do not want to look like a man 13

3. Long sets to cut 19

5. I do abs to lose belly fat 22

6. I am good as I am, I do not need to exercise 25

7. The knees should not go over the toes during a squat 27

8. Swimming, the best sport for the back 30

9. Do not lock your joints at the end of a movement, or you will destroy your joints! 31

10. Bodybuilding is pumping iron. It is not what will make your strong! 33

11. I do not work on machines, I only do functional movements! 36

12. Respecting rest times is necessary or else you will not progress 38

13. Sweating more to work better and to lose more fat! 40

14.	I will be so slow if I do weight training	42
15.	Long sets are only for endurance!	45
16.	I run for long periods and I only do cardio to cut	49
17.	I want a change in 3 to 4 weeks max!	52
18.	Weight training is making me tight	54
19.	You must train every day if you want to progress	56
20.	I will never be good in that because my morphology doesn't allow me to	58
21.	I lack stability	67
22.	Weight training and/ or weightlifting is dangerous and destroys growth (in teens)	69
23.	I am too old to gain muscle	73
24.	CROSSFIT Pull Ups are useless, you might as well do strict pullups	75
25.	The goal is not to be strong in one area, but to be strong everywhere	78
26.	Do not do CrossFit, you will injure yourself!	82
27.	I will lose all my gains if I do not train during a week	85
28.	The deadlift, the king of exercises, essential in bodybuilding	89
29.	Heyyy Patriciiiia! Guess what!? I've bought a new trendy cream which just got out to make cellulite disappear!	92
30.	If I weigh as much, it is because I have big bones.	94

31. The squat recruits as much of the leg muscles possible, you cannot find more complete! 97
32. The Deadlift is more tiring than the Squat! 99
33. A woman must not train like a man 102
34. My knees are painful... certainly due to arthritis ... 104
35. No pain No gain 107
36. Running is dangerous for the knees and for the lower back 110
37. We need to go "harder" on trainings coach, I am not losing weight! There is nothing changing on the scale! 112
38. Heyyyy Jocelyne? Guess what! I invested in my home gym to lose weight! I bought an elliptical bike, and on my first session I've burned 500 calories using it! 114
39. I do cardio before my training session and then I do a big weight training session to cut and build muscle at the same time 116
40. If you take a large grip on your Pull Ups, it will allow you to better target your lats muscles 118
41. It burns so much! I am unable to finish my movement because of lactic acid! 121
42. Improve your muscle gains thanks to pre-exhaustion! 123
43. Base yourself on mind-muscle connection and on sensation to improve your muscle gains! 125
44. A big back for a big bench press! 128

PART 2: Fitness scams: Pointless devices and other hoaxes 133
- 45. The posture shirt 135
- 46. Push Ups board 137
- 47. The legging & the anti-cellulite suction cup 139
- 48. The sweat belt 140
- 49. The weight loss Hula Hoop 143
- 50. The Facial Toner 144
- 51. The double chin mask 145
- 52. The vibration plate 148
- 53. The stepper 150
- 54. The meal replacement shake 152

PART 3: "The VERSUS" 155
- 55. Axle Bar Deadlift VS Olympic Bar Deadlift 157
- 56. Front Squat VS Back Squat (high bar) 162
- 57. Hip Thrust VS Conventional Deadlift 165
- 58. Pull Ups (pronated) VS Chin Ups (supinated) 167
- 59. Reverse Hyperextension VS Back Extension 170
- 60. Good Morning VS Deadlift 173
- 61. Shoulder Press (Barbell) VS Shoulder Press (Dumbbells) 175
- 62. Running on a treadmill VS Running outside 178

63.	Home training VS Gym training 180
64.	Machines VS Free weights 184
65.	Occlusion Training VS Classical Training 186
66.	Overcoming Isometrics VS Yielding Isometrics 189
67.	Dumbbells VS Kettlebells 193
68.	Triceps Extension (bar): Pronated VS supinated ... 196
69.	American Swing VS Russian Swing 198
70.	Front Pulldown vs Behind The Neck Pulldown 200

PART 4: FOR OR AGAINST? 203

71.	The protective foam pad: for or against? 204
72.	Arnold Press: For or against? 206
73.	Squeeze Press (Plate) / Close grip Bench Press (with plates): For or against? 208
74.	Shrug Rotation: For or against? 210
75.	Behind The Neck Press: For or against? 213
76.	Bench Press Suicide Grip: For or against? 215
77.	Weight plate Side Bend: For or against? 217

Introduction

If there is one thing I remember in the world of physical activity and sports, it is that nothing is never all black or white. We can rather find shades of grey. That means that an array of data could differ depending on the context.

This book's ambition is not to deliver you an absolute truth on the world of physical activity and of sports, but rather to push through a deep reflexion whilst making certain notions accessible for the understanding of all.

Through that publication, I am sharing with you my personal experience as a coach and as an international athlete. But also, a personal analysis which derives from numerous exchanges with sports and healthcare professionals. To end with, this publication comes along with a few scientific reviews to back up the enunciated ideas.

I've done my best to remain as objective as possible, but the effort was in vain. And, a book without subjectivity, it's like eating some Kellog's without milk. A bit sad, right?

Am I right? Should you take this book as an absolute truth after having read it? Absolutely not. What is written at a moment in time might as well not be valid tomorrow. Perhaps you will even doubt the veracity of my words. May you agree or not, the mission will be accomplished. Because this book will have allowed you one thing: becoming a better version of yourself as a coach, an athlete, or as a simple passionate individual, by means of critical thinking.

Enjoy your reading!

Partie 1 : Myths and popular beliefs

"To attain the truth, it is needed once in a life to detach yourself from all opinions we have received, and reconstruct once again all the system of our knowledge."
[René Descartes]

1. The Butt Wink is dangerous for your back. Avoid the squat or else you will injure yourself!

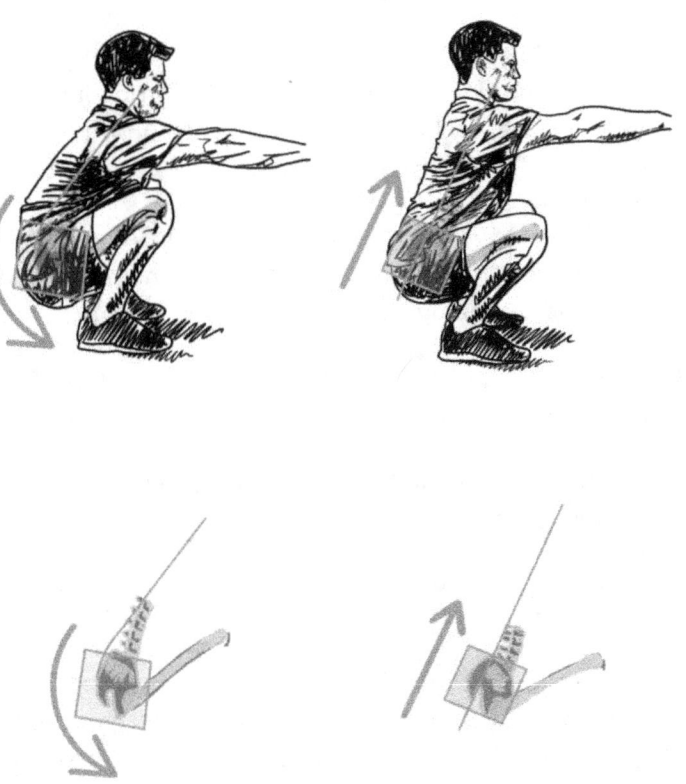

Before looking into whether the Butt Wink is dangerous or not, it is important to understand what a "Butt Wink" is.

In French, the Butt Wink does not really have a definition. It is an anglophone expression which describes the rounding of the spine, and which generally occurs on the squat movement (in the lower position), and specifically, during a full squat.

Now that we know what a "Butt Wink" is, let's look into the popular beliefs and the questionings around it:

Is it dangerous for your back and for your lumbar disks?

The popular belief argues it is. The theory behind it being that an excessive folding could provoke a lesion of lumbar disks[1] throughout time, and that the solution would therefore be to limit our range of motion on the squat.[i]

However, as the spine is locked in a stable position, it is capable of carrying enormous forces. As such, continuing to develop a full squat and obtaining a better tissue recruitment.[ii]

The real problem of the Butt Wink would occur during a loss of the "lumbar curve", and would thus give rise to an injury risk.[iii]

What should be suggested to someone who has a "Butt Wink" on their squat movement?

- Analysis of potential pathologies on behalf of a healthcare professional

- Analysis of potential deficits in terms of mobility before being able to bring up solutions once the source has been found (strengthening of the hip flexors on a flexion, limbering up of the glutes and of the hip rotators, ankle mobility work as well)

- If pain occurs and persists, it is suggested to introduce an alternative to the squat movement which is not problematic. Tempo work to programme or to reprogramme motor control

---

[1] In the spine, we can find 23 discs. 6 in the cervical region, 12 in the thoracic region and 5 in the lumbar region

in every range of motion of the movement is a solution that some healthcare professionals also suggest.

To be taken into account:

On a squat, during the lowering phase, the Butt Wink starts from the bottom. This means that the hip drives the pelvis and then the sacrum on which the lumbar spine rests. The first focus point must therefore be mobility of the lower body. Core engagement is of paramount importance during the movement. In case of a loss or a lack of core engagement, some specialists assert that there is a high risk of developing a herniated disk, or at least, a disk protrusion. Yet, that remains empirical.

However, it is important to keep perspective. In fact, lumbar flexion during a squat is unavoidable even if we try avoiding it[iv]. It is also important to prepare ourselves to receiving constraints on the rachis by realising exercises involving a flexion. Wanting to avoid lumbar flexion at all costs brings along a risk of being weaker during movements involving a flexion, and as such, increasing injury risk.

Conclusion:

It is important to take into account that an injury can occur if there is an excess on the movement and/ or as a result of fatigue accumulation which could lead to a loss of lumbar spine position in the lower position of the squat. Progression on the movement is fundamental. However, the Butt Wink is not problematic in of itself, and has been "demonised" to bring a theoretical explanation to lumbar pain. It is not because someone has a Butt Wink that he cannot perform a squat or that he will be limited forever on the squat movement. To a certain extent, certain pelvic movements are completely normal depending on your anatomy, and some solutions exist to continue developing yourself on the squat movement. That could be through alternative exercises, or mobility works.

2. I want to tone my body but I do not want to look like a man

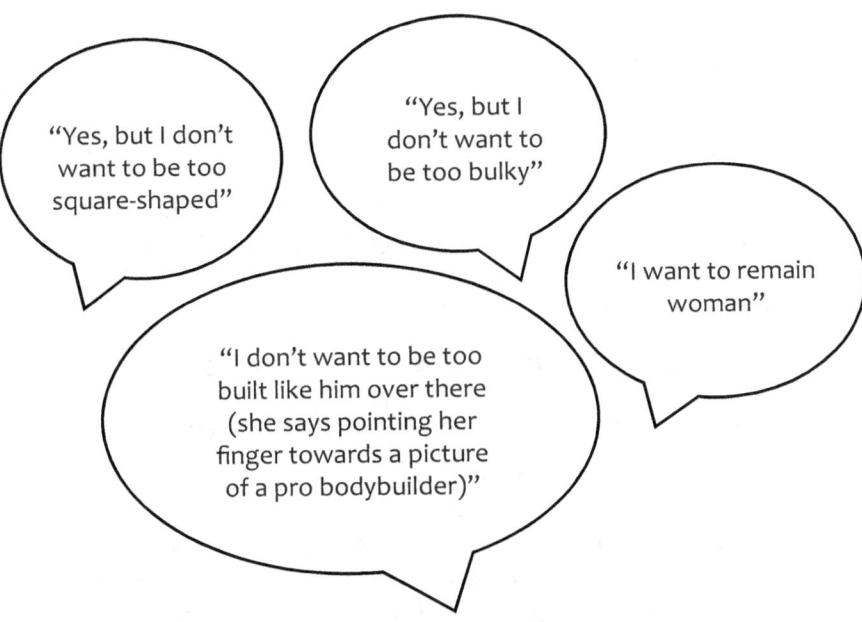

It is hard to count the number of times we have heard this sentence! Perhaps are you even recognising yourself in those words... We are not blaming you!

Above all, it is important to understand that the use of the words "to tone", "toning up", "sculpting your body" are nothing more than commercial expressions which simply mean "BUILDING MUSCLE".

It is to be noted that muscle building will depend on a number of factors for an individual:

- Their sex
- Their genetics[2]
- Their physical activity
- Their age
- ...

"Well, that being said, we still want to know how to remain woman if we decide to get involved in the fitness realm".

No stress! We are getting there!

A man is not a woman and a woman is not a man!

It sounds incredible to read, but it is the truth! (really!?)

Let's start with a relatively simple exercise:

A man and a woman measure the same size, practice the same sports (fitness), have the same sports experience (let's say they practice fitness since 5 years), and have the same age range. The man will always (in the majority of cases at least, with some exceptions) carry more muscle mass than his female counterpart.

Why?

---

[2] We remain here in the "broad lines" by speaking of "genetics", but others factors enter into account such as hormonal genetics and muscular typology for example.

Because certain factors come into play, of which:

- Muscle typology[3]

- Less strength as compared to men (from the start)

Fewer anabolic hormone levels (testosterone) as compared to men. Testosterone is a hormone which plays an important role on health, productivity in sports, wellbeing, as well as libido.

For women, testosterone is produced in smaller amounts by adrenal glands and by ovaries (about 20 times less), whereas for men, the latter is produced in the testicles and in the adrenal glands [45]

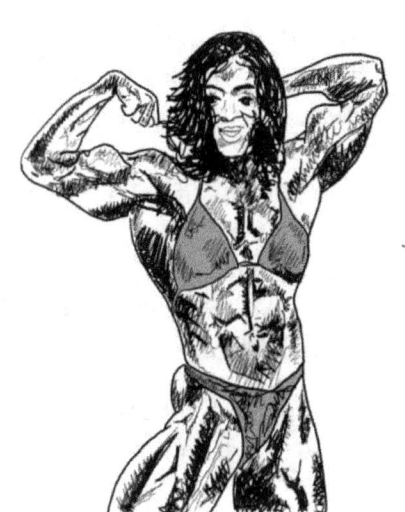

---

[3]   On average, women hold more bodyfat (25 à 30%) and less muscle mass than men (12 à 15%).

[4]   Caution: Testosterone does not explain everything. It is only one factor of development amongst others.

[5]   It would appear that the difference between women and men regarding the level of anabolic hormones is similar to that between a man taking steroid drugs and a man not taking steroid drugs. Regarding athletes taking and not taking steroid drugs, it would appear that we would be between 5 and 29 times the physiological dose.

With all these factors which come into play, this strongly changes the situation, and it means that a woman will not attain the same muscular development than a man (especially when comparing with high level athletes).

"Yes, but at the gym there is a female bodybuilder which is as bulky as a man".

Well.

Note that, prior to attaining a certain level, bodybuilding requires years of practice. And it probably involves a lifestyle much more difficult to bear than for another sport.

In addition, if that supposedly female bodybuilder is "abnormally" muscled (I will come back to the term abnormal that I've just used), well, it is either an exceptional case, or perhaps she simply has used steroid drugs to allow her to attain competition/ career goals, and it is a choice to respect.

I will now come back to the term "abnormally muscled". I do not like the turn that our society is taking at present.

It is only my personal opinion, but our society sees the woman of today as being someone with a slim waist, slim legs, and she must not be muscled because it downgrades the image we have of a woman, and it renders her "too manly".

Do not pay attention to critics.

Do you feel like you are yourself doing CrossFit? THEN DO IT!

Do you feel like you are yourself doing MMA? THEN DO IT!

Do you feel yourself when you practice weightlifting? THEN DO IT!

It is society which is ugly. Not you.

> Conclusion:
>
> Apart if you are a novice in the field and can expect to see results relatively quickly, women should not worry. Physiologically, they are not predisposed to become "ultra-muscled".

« Skinny is not sexy. Health Is. »

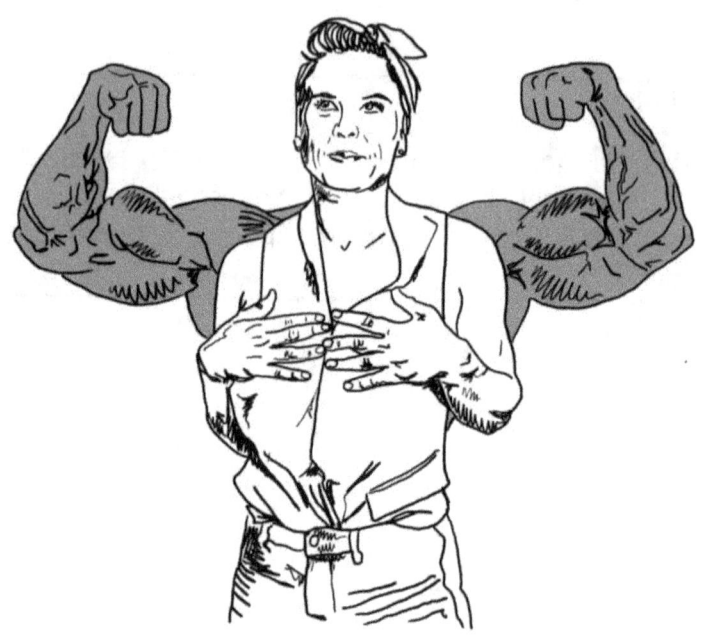

3. Long sets to cut

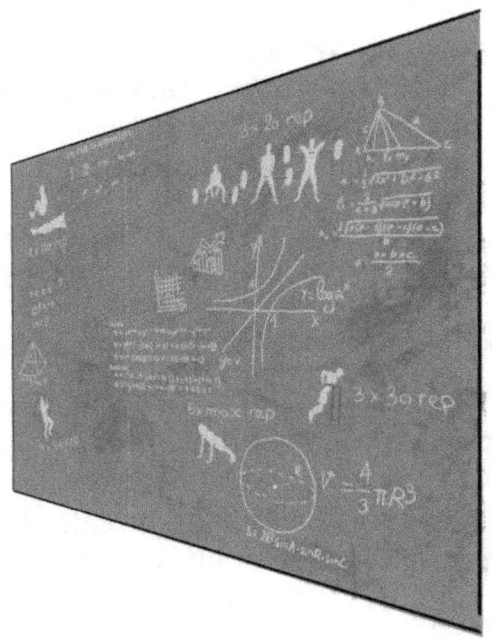

Another idea widespread in the fitness world! And yet...

The popular belief being that if we do a lot of repetitions, it will exclusively be to lose fat ("to cut"), and it would allow to be leaner visually. On the contrary, doing sets with less repetitions would allow to put on more muscle mass and be stronger.

But, is that really the case?

There is no miracle recipe. If you want to be "more shredded" and have a better muscle definition, you will need to lose fat!

To have more muscle definition, you must therefore have a lower bodyfat percentage. It is not because you are feeling that your muscle is burning during an effort that you are actually burning bodyfat.

The work to be done will therefore essentially involve what you put on your plate by implementing a caloric deficit (the caloric deficit occurring as you consume less energy than you are burning through physical activities or that your energy expenditure linked to physical activities increases).

To add more content regarding weight training, carrying weights increases excess post-exercise oxygen consumption (EPOC[6]). Cela est dû au stress métabolique que la musculation impose à l'organisme.

Training at a high intensity[7] with high loads multiple times per week is all the more useful as it simultaneously recruits muscles and neurological transmission, favouring not only muscle definition[8] but also an improved coordination.[vi]

---

[6]   EPOC: excess post-exercise oxygen consumption. That effect remains minimal nonetheless. Hence the importance of having a diet which concords with your goals.

[7]   It is important to take a step back concerning intensity. Intensity is relative depending on the individual, Progression is an important step in the process. Being at "100%" in your mental and physical capacities during each training session is not possible.

[8]   More defined musculature: commercial term. This means a musculature "with a lower body fat percentage".

Conclusion:

Long sets are useful for goals other than weight loss. Concentrate yourself on having a diet suited to your needs and to your lifestyle. Build confidence on the loads you are using, continue progressing, and don't be afraid of heavy loads!

5. I do abs to lose bodyfat

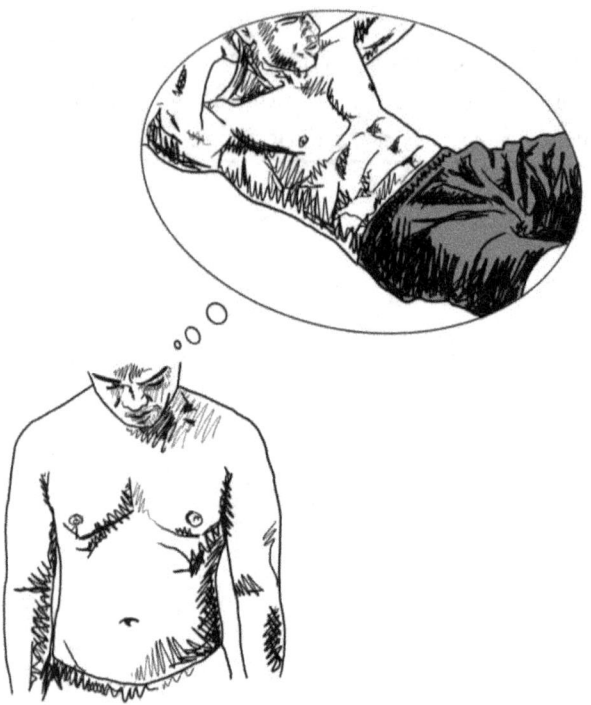

Don't laugh, it is nowadays still possible to find people who put forward this kind of absurdity.

Is it their fault? Clearly not. As a coach, it is of my duty to battle against such misconceptions.

Unfortunately, it is impossible to specifically target where fat loss occurs.

Nonetheless, it is possible to take charge of yourself by:

- Performing multi-joint exercises
- Putting a caloric deficit in place[9]
- Arming yourself with patience and discipline

In fact, multi-joint exercises will allow to involve more muscles, and as such, burn more calories. To give you an idea, a Sumo Deadlift will burn more calories than a Biceps Curl.

Note:

Although that is completely empirical[10], certain coaches or sports professionals assert that with the help of an extreme training protocol (often associated with a very high volume), it could be possible to target where fat loss occurs. In a situation in which fat loss would be looked for, the technology of cryolypolisis, a cold treatment aimed at destroying fat cells, would allow to target fat loss on certain parts of the body. However, the effect remains very small.

---

[9] The image put on the article is just an indication related to BMI (Body Mass Index). It is placed in order to have a "general" idea.

[10] Which is only based on experience, on observation, and not on a theory or on reasoning (The Robert Dictionary)

> Conclusion:
>
> According to current research[11], we cannot target fat loss via physical activity in a precise way. However, let's keep in mind that sport evolves every single day, and the we must not cease to question ourselves.

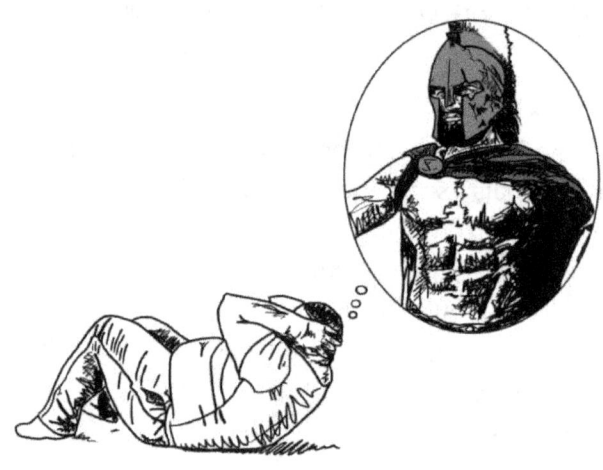

---

[11] A research entitled "Effect of combined resistance and endurance exercise training on regional fat loss" issued from "The journal of Sports Medicine and Physical Fitness" made me hesitant regarding the discourse around targetable fat loss. After having read the research and having exchanged with other professionals in the field, we have agreed that it is not possible to target fat loss in an "ultra precise" way. But that study opens up new perspectives on fat loss in the realm of sports.

6. I am good as I am, I do not need to exercise

So, that one... It is so ludicrous that it deserves the Golden Globe!

Scoop of the year: The practice of sports is not only reserved to the goal of losing weight. There are so many benefits that it is hard to cite them all!

- **On a social level:**

- Creates friendships, encounters around a physical activity involving a passion
- Instils notions such as team spirit, mutual aid and respect

- **On a psychological level:**[vii]

- Fight against anxiety
- Increases the brain's oxygenation. That means increased intellectual performance (well, where is the cliché of the jacked guy without a brain?)
- Allows to secret endorphins, wellbeing hormone which brings along a pleasure sensation

- **On a physiological level:**

- Improves the cardio-vascular system (yes, the heart is also a "cardiac" muscle)
- Contributes to the retention of muscle mass
- Helps with transit
- Improves respiratory capabilities

- Serves as a prevention tool against joint problems

- Helps to solidify bones (increases bone mineral density)

- Stimulates the immune system

Conclusion:

Sports (or physical activity) brings you substantial advantages to be healthy.

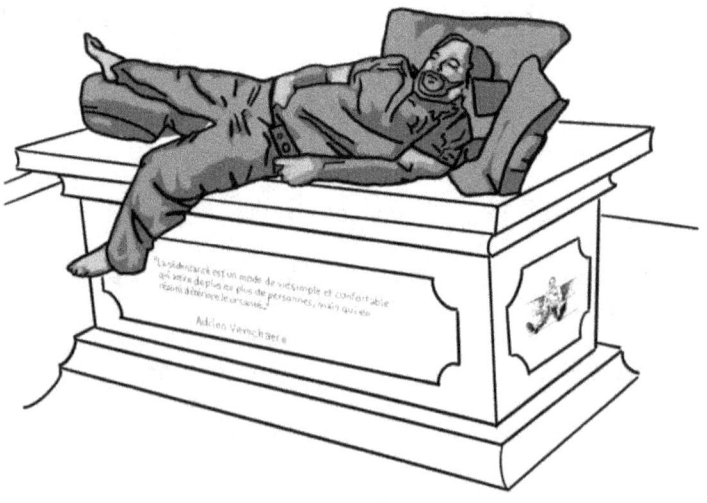

7. Les genoux ne doivent pas dépasser les orteils au squat

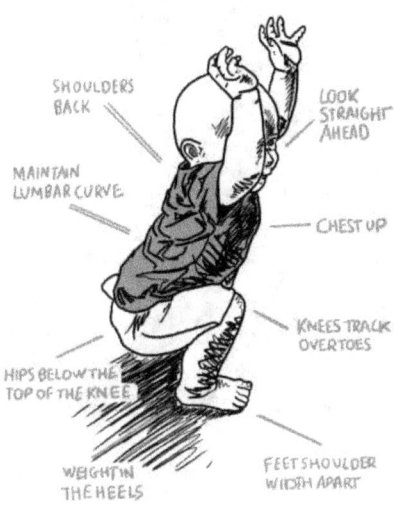

Although that myth is increasingly less widespread, it still exists and it is time to completely annihilate it!

For long, the instruction "Do not let the knees pass in front of the tip of your toes" has been maintained. The idea being to reduce the pressure we could put on the knees, and so, on the long term, bring along an injury risk.

Although the idea makes sense, it does not mean that it is a good one nonetheless. The squat is a natural movement.

Since our very young age, we instinctively adopt that position.

In a number of Asian countries, crouching (Full Squat) is totally normal, and it is a position used to wait, eat, work… By the way, this position is popularised by the term "Asian squat".

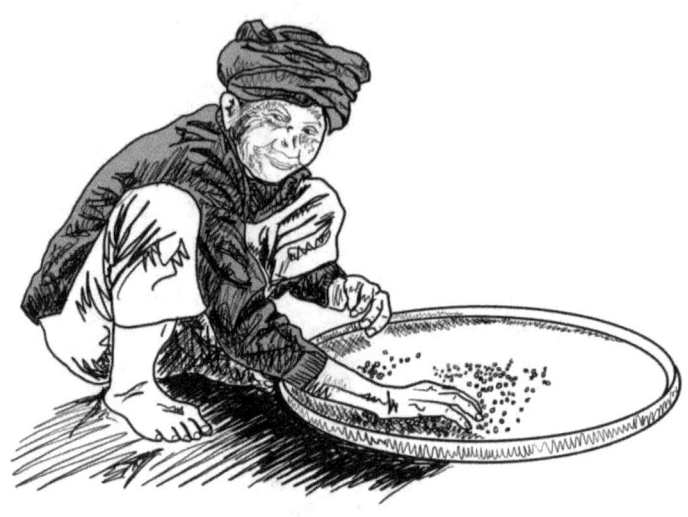

Apparently, from a theoretical standpoint, Western education and cultural norms are what led us to forget that resting position via the use of chairs, tables, toilets, which imply a 90-degrees sitting position.

To get back to the squat in weight training, it is totally natural and logical to perform a full squat with the knees going over the toes.

The real risk of not wanting to let the knees voluntarily pass forward the tip of your toes is to bring more tension in the lower back as well as in the hips.

The factors which will ensure that your knees are placed at a certain position/ range of motion during a squat will depend on:

- Your flexibility (principally of the hip and of the ankles)

- Of the length of your segments

By the way, thinking a little bit, as we climb up and then go back down the stairs, the knees pass in front the tip of our toes, right? Another example remains the practice of weightlifting with athletes carrying impressive loads whilst having their knees which go over the tip of their toes. By the way, A study which got out in 2012 glorifies the Full Squat, and it even demonstrates that the problem isn't the squat exercise *per se*, but rather its execution.[viii]

> Conclusion:
> Having the knees which go over the toes is a natural movement during the squat. There is no need to worry about it.

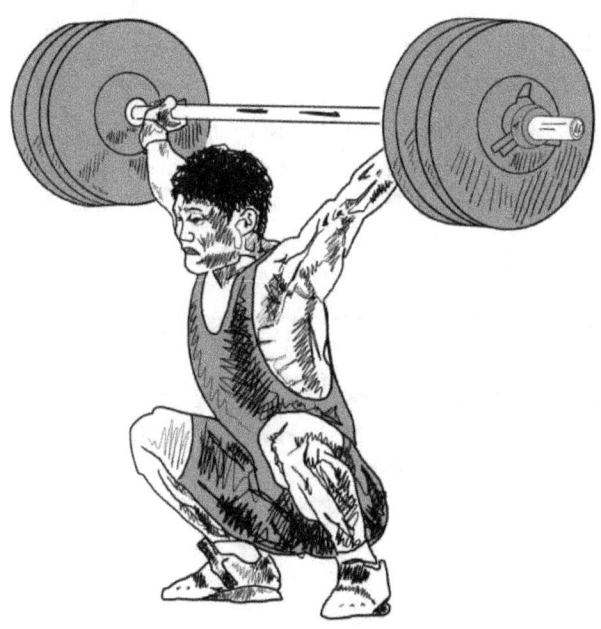

8. La natation, le meilleur sport pour le dos

The popular belief holds that the best sport the back would be swimming.

But what is it really all about?

We suppose that this belief comes from the fact that aquatic activity would allow to avoid "shock waves".

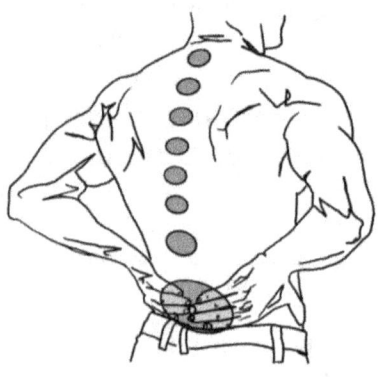

However, a study realised on teenagers (medium age of 14-15 years old) demonstrated that biking and walking were more effective than swimming as it relates to back pain![ix]

The goal here is not to spit on swimming. Far from that. Exercises involved in aquatic sports (e.g. aquagym) have proven good results for back pain of the "lumbago"[12] type. However, they have not demonstrated more results than terrestrial activities.[x]

Conclusion:

Do what you enjoy doing. Swimming is not the most effective to avoid back pain. Nonetheless, if you enjoy practicing swimming, then go enjoy yourself!

---

12   Lumbago: term which refers to "lumbar pain"

9. Do not lock your joints at the end of a movement, or you will destroy your joints!

It is an instruction that we still regularly hear nowadays, and it is not necessarily a bad one in certain sports situations. What matters is to contextualise.

Consequently, here, I will not speak of:

- Active range of motion (the fact of keeping your muscle under tension)

- Of eventual elbow, shoulder, knee pathologies...

- Of hyperlaxity

Illustrating with a counter-argument this type of statement is the best to be done:

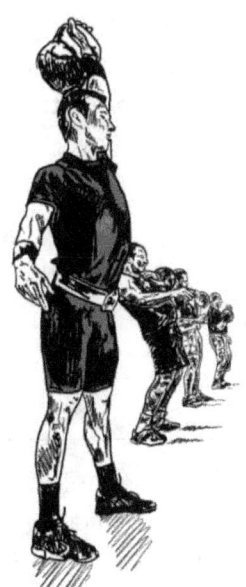

- Do you think that a weight lifter would be capable of maintaining a load above his head if he wasn't locking out his joints? Personally, I prefer stopping the suspense right now and tell you that if the weight lifter did not lock out his joints, it is very likely for him to see a few hundreds of kilos fall on his head.

- Do you think a kettlebell sport athlete would be capable of validating his repetitions if he didn't lock out his joints? I would also add that the volume performed during certain competitions, and that the prescribed loads still hasn't led athletes such as Denis Vasilev[13] or Stéphane

Dogman[14] retire from their sports. If it was fundamentally dangerous, this sport would not exist.

- Do you think that carrying a schoolbag (which constitutes an additional load) whilst waiting for your bus is done with a slight flexion to preserve your joints?

The extension of the joint is necessary, and it comes in handy in certain rest situations (sports-related or not). Whether it is to do pauses between repetitions or to validate certain repetitions during a competition.

Conclusion:

Before demonising locking out the joints by putting forward that it is synonymous with injury, it is important to contextualise. Pathologies or certain training methods put aside, locking out your joints is a totally normal process to rest between the repetitions of a set and to validate your repetitions in a competition for certain sports.

---

13   Denis Vasilev is a multiple world-champion in kettlebell sport

14   Stéphane Dogman is a French kettlebell sport athlete and also a selector of the French team in that sport. He is considered to be a precursor of that discipline in his country

10. Bodybuilding is pumping iron. It is not what will make your strong!

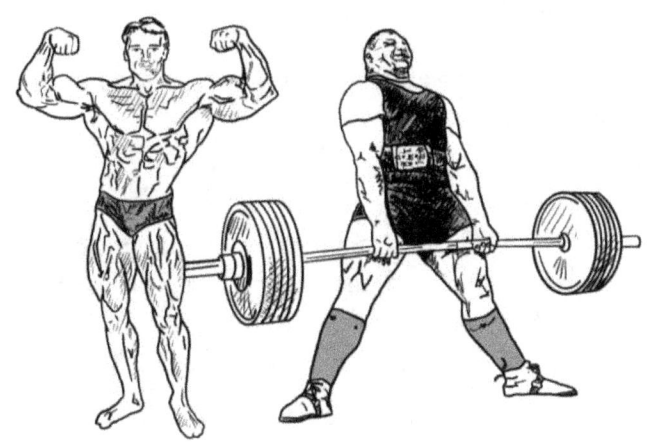

The term "Gonflette" (French expression which could be translated by "pumping iron") is still atrociously pejorative when it is mentioned in the bodybuilding space.

But what is bodybuilding?

Bodybuilding is weight training which is geared towards "sculpting" the body. An art which consists of developing your muscle mass whilst holding on the least possible body fat for an aesthetic purpose.

Consequently, bodybuilding's first goal is not to develop your maximal strength.

Strength, on its part, depends on multiple factors:

- Muscle typology[15]

- Muscle fibre length

- Muscle fibre width

- Motor units synchronisation[16]

- The capacity of recruitment of a certain number of motor units in the least possible time

- The physiological cross-sectional area[xi][17]

Because individuals practising bodybuilding essentially work on structural and non-nervous factors, this explains why their strength is less developed than for a powerlifter[18], despite the bodybuilder appearing "more voluminous".

---

[15] Muscle typology: percentage of slow-twitch and fast-twitch muscle fibres.

[16] A motor unit is made by a motor neuron located in the spinal cord, its prolongation (axon) which goes through the peripheral nerve and the totality of muscle fibres which it innervates.

[17] In muscle physiology, the physiological cross-sectional area (PCSA) is the cross-sectional surface of a muscle perpendicular to its fibres, generally at its biggest point. It is typically used to describe the contraction properties of pennate muscles. According to a study, there would be a better correlation at total muscular volume.

[18] Powerlifter: Terms used to describe an individual practising powerlifting. Powerlifting being a strength sports discipline of which the goal is to carry the heaviest possible load on the Back Squat, the Bench press and the Deadlift with an Olympic Barbell.

> Conclusion:
>
> Carrying heavy loads will allow stimulating nervous factors to improve your maximal strength. However, putting on muscle mass does not necessarily mean that we need to carry heavy loads as we take the risk of less isolating our muscles, and as such, not attain the initially desired aesthetic goal. Every individual is different be it with regards to the adaptation of their nervous system, a concern related to strength development... Hence, do what you enjoy doing according to your feelings!

11. I do not work on machines, I only do functional movements!

We've already all heard it! That might be in a fitness gym, a CrossFit box, or even with friends whilst sharing your last PRs around a shaker!

Today, the word functional is used in every possible way. So, how to find your way through that?

The popular belief would want the word "functional" to be synonymous with bodyweight training, free weights training (barbells, sandbags, kettlebells, dumbbells…) and suspension training (e.g. TRX). Essentially, everything which does not involve training with machines.

The fact behind it being that, from the start, our muscles have many functions, including an important one: MOVING!

That means that it is impossible (exceptional cases and pathologies put aside) to have "non-functional" muscles.

If that was the case, they would be of no use (apart from… decorating perhaps?)

Beware!

The fact of using certain exercises rather than others by diligently choosing the material with which you will train depending on the targeted goal will be crucial. Once again, it all depends on the context!

To be taken into account:

Science[xii] looked into functional training. To this day, there is no universally agreed upon definition of functional training. These trainings tend to develop the same benefits which are already induced by "traditional" programmes.

> Conclusion:
>
> The fact that you are working with machines does not mean that you are not building functional muscle. Muscle possesses many functions of which knowing how to mobilise yourself in your environment. Simply pay attention to the context when choosing your exercises.

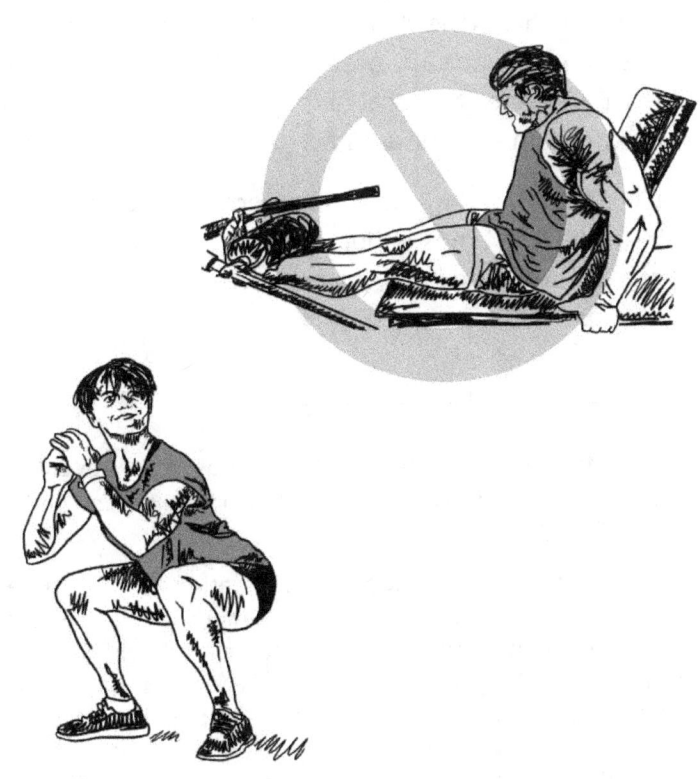

12. Respecting rest times is necessary or else you will not progress

Here again, contextualising is required (decidedly, this word constantly comes around!).

I've always thought that when we ask quite a general question to a coach, a good coach would simply reply:

"It depends"

So, I will provide some examples:

When I prepared myself for the 2019 marathon world championship (One Arm Jerk 24kg) in kettlebell sport[19], rest time was essential in order to add in more sets in a same timeframe since the goal here is reach a maximum number of repetitions in a set timeframe.

In contrast, in the case of hypertrophy or even in that of strength, rest times should be longer in order to let enough time to the body to correctly recover to accomplish the prescribed sets.[20]

---

[19] Marathon kettlebell sport: it is a 60-minutes event during which it is not permitted to put the kettlebell on the ground under penalty of disqualification.

[20] Fearful of an erroneous interpretation, I would rather bring an explication via this end of page annotation: once again, it all depends on the context. If the goal is to target metabolic stress within the framework of hypertrophy, with methods such as the Legeard method or breakdown training, for example, there will be a value in compressing or suppressing rest times. These are interesting intensification methods when time is a limiting factor in our trainings.

What we should remember is that, depending on the context, rest times are not a key factor. If we are in the field of endurance, this allows to measure our progress. What matters is to not fall into excess by, for example, taking huge rest times for moderately intense efforts.

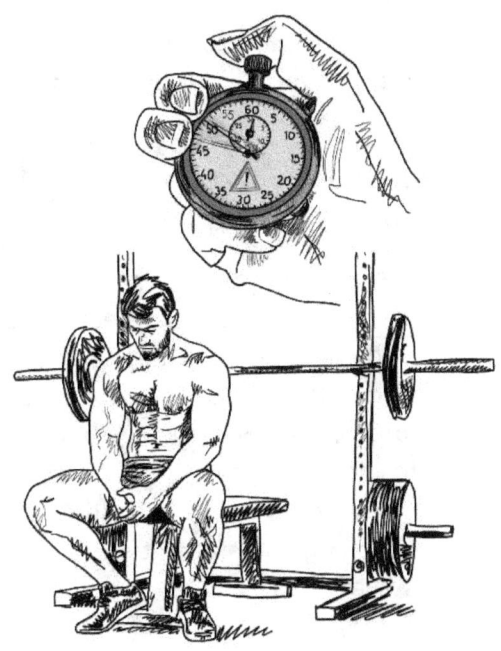

Conclusion:

Put aside certain specific situations linked to metabolic stress, rest times are not essential to progress as long as we correctly define the context and that we do not fall in an extreme depending on the effort to be done (to not spend 3 hours training for example). Every individual is different and every individual has their own capacity of adaptation.

13. Sweating more to work better and to lose more fat!

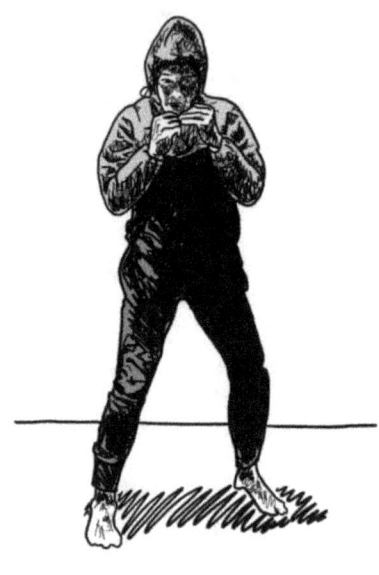

OK, no time to dither[21]. Sweating more does not mean that you will burn more calories!

Also, it is not because you sweat a lot that you have worked better.

Sweat occurs when your body has to regulate its temperature. This allows to cool down the skin.

And that goes with another point that we still hear: your bodyfat does not transform itself into muscle. This is physiologically impossible. Bodyfat is "burned" inside the body. Et ça rejoint un autre point que l'on entend encore : Votre graisse ne se transforme pas en muscle. It does not transform itself nor is it evacuated under the form of sweat.

To be taken into account:

We do not burn more calories by sweating, but by thermoregulating. This can turn out to be dangerous on the long term. The more we maintain an intensity under heat, the more the difficulty increases.

---

[21] Using detours, red herrings, to avoid giving a clear response, to delay the decision-making process (The Robert Dictionary)

> Conclusion:
>
> Sweat is a biological response of the body which just allows the latter to refresh itself.

14. I will be slow if I do weight training

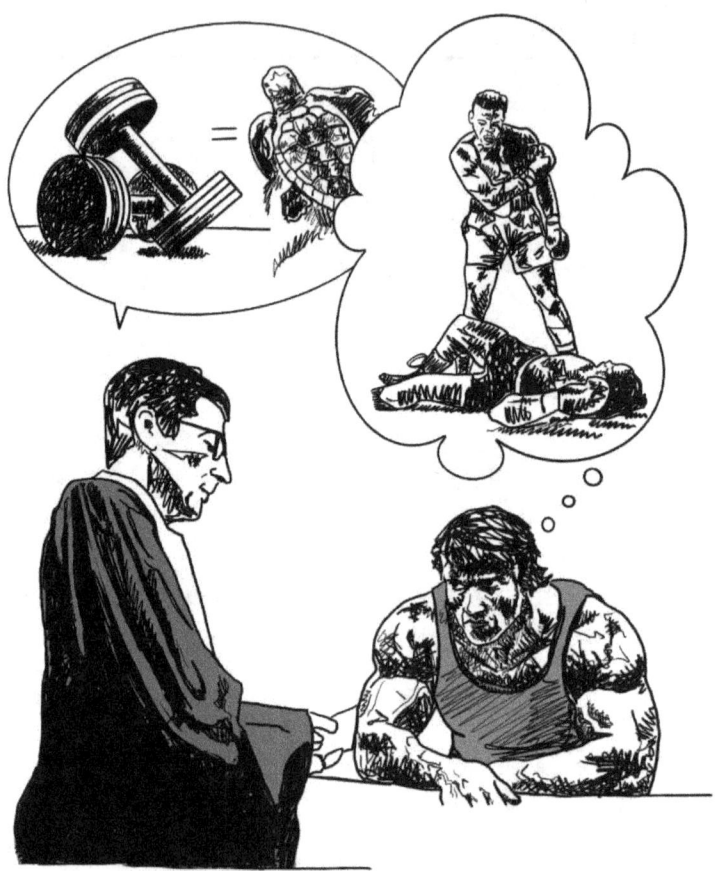

That cliché, I heard it many times when I played basketball before turning myself to kettlebell sport. And I am convinced that I am not the only one to have heard it!

And, it is an argument which continuously, but wrongfully, comes back. Be it in the world of running or of other endurance-type sports.

Why is this false?

If we look at certain sports disciplines, a decisive factor is to run a certain distance within the minimum amount of time possible. Speed is therefore important.

Many studies (on running) have shown that a strength-style training has a positive state to improve running economy[22],[xiii]

Let's go back to a simple example from True Fitness Knowledge[23]:

"If during a race, your mean strength applied in the ground is of 2000 Newtons per stride and that your maximal strength is of 4000 Newtons, then your effort is at 50% of your maximum capacity. However, by improving your force at 5000 Newtons thanks to an appropriate training and by keeping your initial intensity at 50%, your mean force applied in the ground is now of 2500 Newtons per stride. So, logically, you will advance more rapidly and your performance will be improved via a better running economy."

---

[22] Running economy: is defined as the ability of an individual to efficiently move on the energetic realm (serval.unil.ch)

[23] True Fitness Knowledge is the name given to a physical trainer working since many years. He is graduated from a Master 2 (5-years post high school) in Science of Sports and of Nutrition from the "UFR STAPS de Montpellier" and from a Master's Degree (4-years post high school) in Physical and Sports Education from the University of Sherbrooke (UdeS) in Canada. He is also renowned for his informative articles on sport published on the Instagram app.

To be completely transparent with you, it turns out that it is a bit more complex than the example given above. Other mechanical factors enter into account:

- The slope of installation of the strength

- The total length of application of the strength

Both these factors can influence performance without increasing maximum strength.

However, it is clear that to improve your speed, improving your strength is a factor which could improve sporting performances. Therefore, there can be a stake for realising a speed block after a strength block.

> Conclusion:
>
> Although that is not the unique factor involved in speed development, weight lifting and strength training are useful steps if you want to perform in endurance sports.

15. Long sets are only for endurance!

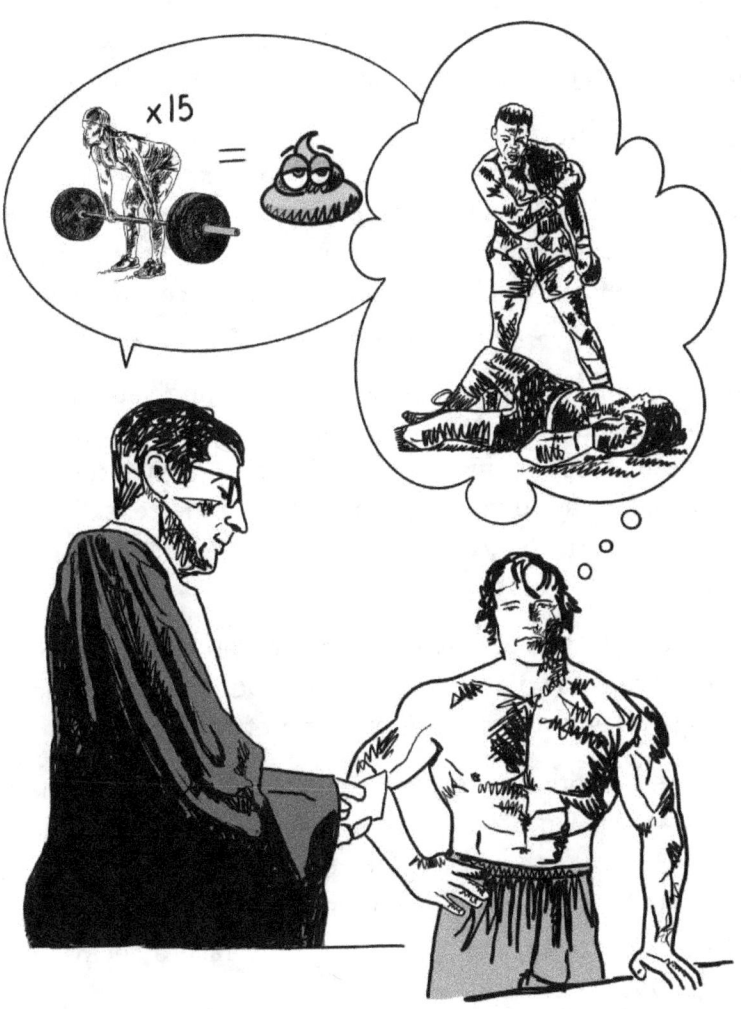

NO! It is partly for endurance!

What do we consider being a long set? Well, I admit that it is quite subjective. We do not all have to agree, but in general, we consider that performing 12 repetitions or more constitutes a long set.

We tend to believe that performing long sets will not allow us to build muscle. On the contrary, these would only be intended to cut. In fact, the fault of a theory positing that that by working with long sets we would only recruit slow-twitch muscle fibres[24] which are not intended to "grow in an optimal way".

Amongst the numerous studies done on long sets in weight training, a study[xiv] conducted in 2009 shows that long sets of 18-20 repetitions performed at 65% of one's RM (4 sets) did not lead to significant differences compared to shorter sets of 8-10 repetitions performed at 80-85% of one's RM (for 4 sets as well) regarding hypertrophy.

In addition to the abovementioned research, other research papers have shown basic notions to favour hypertrophy linked to long sets and volume in terms of repetitions[xv] :

- 5 repetitions and above seem to be a good foundation to build muscle
- 10 to 30 sets per week for a same muscle group seems to be a good range for muscle gains
- A range of 1 to 4 reps far from failure seems to be optimal to build muscle

---

[24] Slow-twitch muscle fibres = Type I fibres. Fast-twitch muscle fibres = Types II fibres

- It is possible to build muscle at a low intensity (less than 60% of your RM) just as it is possible to build muscle at a high intensity (above 60% of your RM[25]). The most important would be to get close to muscle failure.

Apart from that fact, long sets can represent a real challenge. That can be interesting for certain sports disciplines to test the mental abilities of the athlete.

By the way, a programme created by Rory Patrick popularised under the name of "The 20 reps Squat programme" of which the goal is precisely to maximise your gains and your strength by challenging you session after session on long sets.

Nonetheless, a word of caution on using training variables wisely by paying attention to your anthropometry, your level, and by carefully choosing your exercises.

---

[25] RM = Repetition maximum.

> Conclusion:
>
> Long sets are not "just for endurance". They do favour muscle growth and they will seriously put your mental capacities to the test.

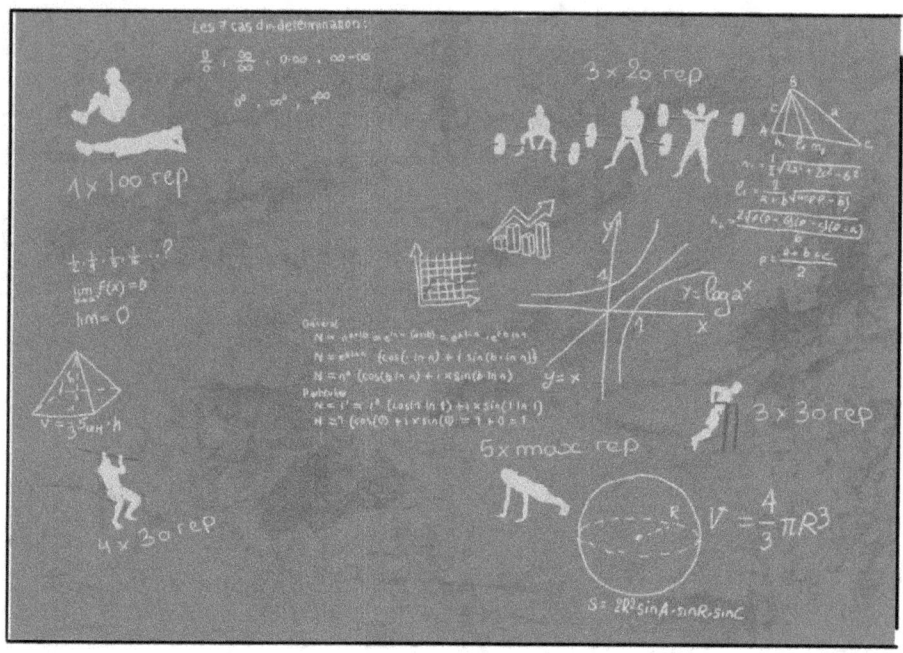

16. I run for long periods and I only do cardio to cut

How many times have I not passed in front of the cardio space in a gym?

How many times have I not passed by the same people, at the same times, on the same days, doing the same cardio session with the same intensity on the machines used?

And unfortunately, in the majority of cases, these same individuals did not obtain the desired results after a few months of practice.

A lack of information and a popular belief which posits that cardio will allow you to rapidly "cut" are to blame.

This is false, and the solution can be summed up in two factors:

- Intensity

- Time

First of all, we must understand that weight loss is related to the caloric deficit. This involves a reduction of your caloric intake (via diet) or an increase of your energy expenditure.

Then, "cardio" is a tool, but it is not mandatory for weight loss (it still remains a major asset for health, which is important to specify). Nonetheless, if you want to lose weight by using that type of tool to achieve your goals, you must understand that energy expenditure is dependent on intensity per unit of time.

A special mention on H.I.I.T.:

According to a study published in 2011, HIIT (High Intensity Interval training) proved itself as being much more interesting for fat loss than longer sessions of cardio at low intensity. In fact, this study has been able to observe a non-negligible decrease of abdominal and subcutaneous fat loss after 15 weeks of training by comparing individuals practising HIIT and individuals practising cardio at low intensity.[xvi]

The reasons being that the intensity that we put within our training bring along improvements on multiple physiological aspects (hormone release, blood pressure improvements, the body continues to burn fat cells 48h after training...).

Multiple possible HIIT methods such as TABATAS (well-known in CrossFit), sprints, training circuits, and more, exist... These principally involve alternating between one/ many exercises with a high or maximum intensity and defined rest times.

There would be a tendency to increasingly recommend HIIT for the purpose of obesity prevention.

Let's here take into account that this is only one study and that I must add a few clarifications. First of all, nothing has changed regarding the abovementioned words. The caloric deficit remains the foundation for weight loss.

Then, H.I.I.T. starts at 90% of your VO2 max[26]. We are therefore very far from commercial trends which leave us assuming the contrary with gentle training circuits. This type of effort is not recommended for novices.

---

[26]   VO2max: maximal oxygen consumption.

Finally, post-training fat loss (related to physiological responses) is not magical[xvii]. On average, we are referring to a loss of about 30 to 70 calories[xviii]. If we speak of a compounding effet, there could be a stake, but this is to be evalutaed with the external contexts surrounding the individual under supervision (example: recovery capacity).

> Conclusion:
>
> HIIT (High Intensity Interval Training) and low intensity endurance exercises are simply just tools favouring weight loss. The most important element remains weight loss. Working on your "cardio" has substantial health benefits. It notably contributes to longevity.

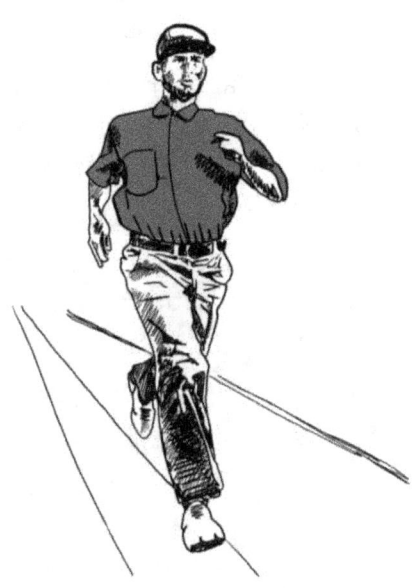

17. I want a change in 3 to 4 weeks max!

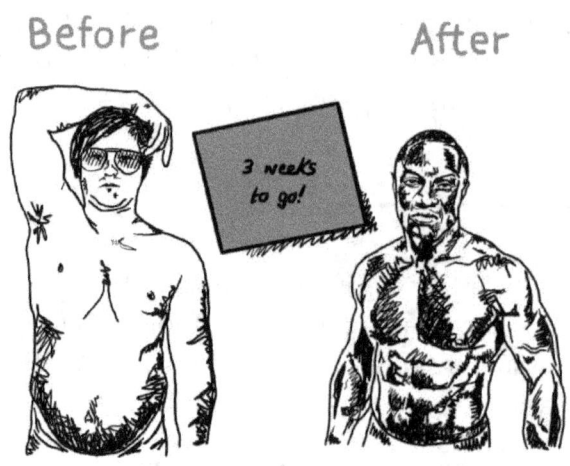

"How long will it take to see initial results"

"I'm leaving on holidays soon, I have 4 weeks to change"

I believe that every coach has already heard that at least once in their life! And I think that a good coach which is faced with a client asking him that question should simply answer "it depends".

And that especially in the case where we do not know the individual questioning us on goals that they would like to obtain.

Every individual is different. This is undeniable. Amongst the factors[27] which will possibly induce faster results than for others, we can mention:

---

[27] The main factors are cited, but others of course exist, such as pathologies and medical history.

- Genetic potential

- Lifestyle (sedentary or not)

- Training frequency

- Diet

And more! By the way, that is why some quit after a few weeks. Because they are imagining results by projecting themselves too rapidly.

Do you earn the same salary with 0 as compared to 5 years of experience?

Were you the same individual 10 years ago?

Well, with sports, it's the same idea! You must keep patience and persevere to attain your goals. You must have a long-term vision and congratulate yourself for achieving each little goal which pushes you towards attaining your vision.

Conclusion:

Every individual is different. Be patient in attaining your goal and believe in yourself.

18. Weight training is making me tight

It is an argument I am hearing less than I used to (which is a good thing), but I still hear it!

It is important to know that it is a myth! On the contrary, weight training and flexibility are not incompatible.

A literature review on excentric work (one of the working phases we can note on a movement) would should a gain in terms of flexibility[xix]

Also, during full range of motion movements, you are mobilising your muscles, your joints and your tendons in a repetitive manner. The fact of adding a load to perform the exercise leads to a wider movement.

Although the addition of loading is sometimes a controversial topic for certain coaches as it does not reflect a natural way to improve a movement, research confirmed that similar improvements are seen between healthy individuals performing exercises with a full range of motion and individuals performing static stretches[xx].

Nevertheless, the advice to be given would be to take into account the adherence of the individual under supervision. This does not mean that everyone should thus use a method with additional loads to improve their flexibility. That just means that it is a method which could suit certain individuals wishing to improve their flexibility.

Conclusion:

Performing weight training movements with a full range of motion can improve flexibility.

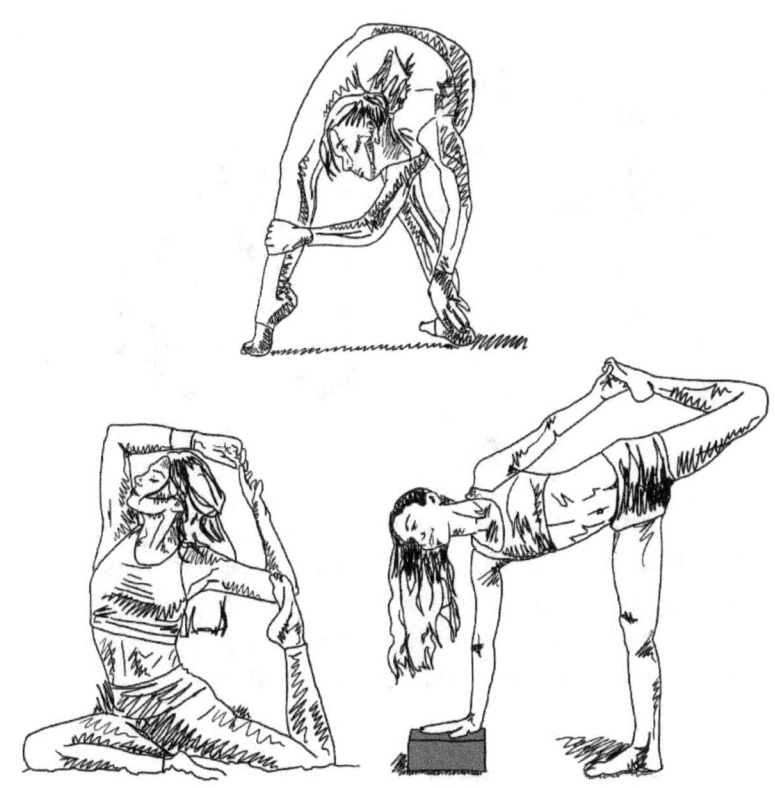

19. You must train every day if you want to progress

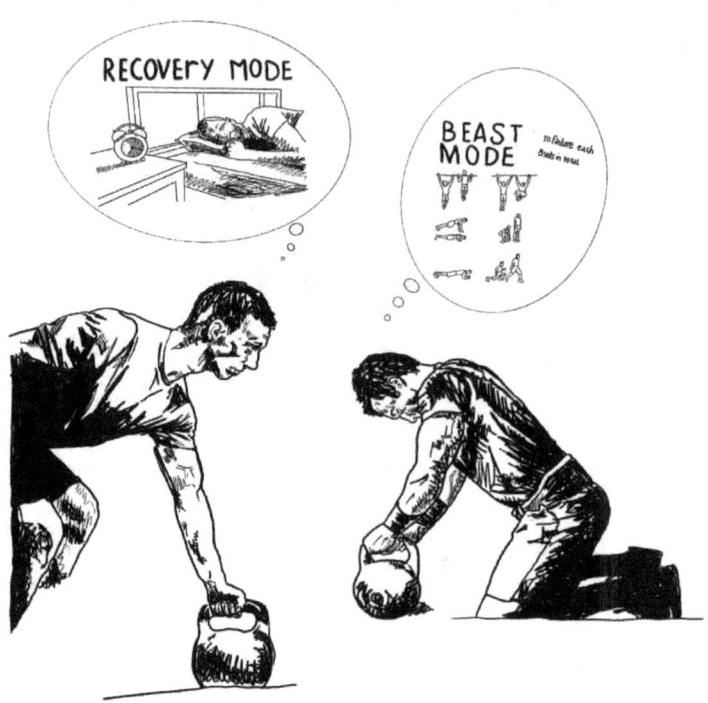

That is completely false. It is a mistake which can lead to overwork and injury if recovery factors are not respected. On the contrary, this does not mean that training every day during a certain period of time will lead to an injury. The desire to train everyday sometimes comes from bigorexia[28].

---

[28] Bigorexia is a dependency to physical activity which involves individuals who became dependent following an excessive practice of sport. (Wik. Def)

Hence the importance of introducing "deload" phases (periods during which training intensity and/ or volume is reduced to favour recovery) in your training programmes.

Nonetheless, although the quote "better a little bit than nothing" takes on its meaning in the realm of physical exercise, it will be very difficult to attain notable long-term results by training less than three times per week with no regularity if you are already involved in sports and have a minimum of experience.

In fact, scientific research allowed noticing that training once or twice per week was not enough to continue progressing. That being said, three trainings per week do indeed allow that.[xxi]

Conclusion:

Training every day is not the ultimate solution if you want to progress (although that might be possible for a given period). If you want to continue progressing overtime, you should train at least three times per week with that frequency being regular. Below that training frequency, you will stagnate (on the long term).

20. I will never be good in that because my morphology doesn't allow me to.

> "Yes, but with my long femurs it is normal for me to be less strong on a squat, so it is useless for me to put efforts into that movement!"

> "Yes, but with my long arms it is normal for me to not be strong on the bench press."

This could lead to confusion. It is therefore important to elucidate the basis of this thought:

Yes, clearly, morphology influences sports performance. It would even be wise to speak of "anthropometry"[29] rather than of morphology alone, and of the analysis we could derive from it (it is too reductionist to only focus on lever arms). Then, it involves knowing what is the between anthropometry and the targeted goal (Development of maximal strength on a specific movement? Muscle growth?); amongst the different research studies conducted, many interesting articles address the topic.

---

[29] Anthropometry being a measurement technique for the human body and its different parts. In another vein, we can sometimes hear the term morpho-anatomy (popularised term).

A study[xii] would have demonstrated the relationship between morphology and performance on the Back squat, the Bench Press and the Deadlift. As follow are the factors which we can derive from this study:

-      Having a thicker torso would allow to have better performances in the three powerlifting movements (Squat, Bench and Deadlift).

-      The smaller the size of the shins, the more advantageous it is for the Squat and the Bench Press. What is surprising is that long femurs do not seem to be a problem to perform on these movements.

This gives us food for thought regarding the influence of morphology and the popular belief on long femurs on the squat. Let's pursue the train of thought a little bit further…

Another research study[xxiii] had for goal to evaluate to what extent ankle mobility and the ratios of the length of the chest, the legs and the calves are responsible for torso incline on the high bar back squat in trained athletes. The conclusion of the study was interesting because it explained that to avoid being too inclined forward on the squat, it was important to work on your ankle mobility. Regarding the theory of long femurs, it would appear that for two individuals of the same build, the one who has a less developed ankle mobility, even of just 10°, would have a same torso incline in comparison to someone having femurs 5cm longer.[xxiv]

Is that all? Of course not!

It is maybe not your case (and that's for the better!). But it is not the first time that we hear that the Bench Press with a full range of motion is to be banned in the case where we have a flat rib cage and long arms, or else we would risk injuring ourselves.

In the case of the development of maximal strength on this movement, it is true that having a large ribcage and short arms seems like a considerable advantage. However, in the perspective of muscle gain, reducing the range of motion does not appear to be the best solution. On the contrary, a greater range of motion leads to more muscle hypertrophy[xxv]. Regarding injuries, progressivity remains the fundamental foundation for different bodily structures to adapt. If that one is respected, then there should not be any problems!

Come on, another one! During a competition of the 2020 CrossFit Games (30 high level athletes), an investigation was conducted on the 1000m rowing "for time"[30]. The goal of this investigation was to answer some questions, and of these ones, there was one which caught my attention:

"Do tall athletes obtain the best scores?"

It is important to specify that the goal of the investigation was to question ourselves on the relevancy of the associations morpho-anatomy/ performance with regards to high level CrossFit athletes. It would appear that the results only show a medium correlation between the size of female athletes and performances. For men, there just appears to be a medium correlation.[xxvi]

Although science is not an opinion, it remains important to not jump to premature conclusions, but to consider these studies as "an indication". At least, this allows having evidence of a higher level as compared to pure speculation.

---

[30] For time means "as fast as possible"

As an international competitor, I am lucky to be able to exchange with physical trainers and with other competitors of different backgrounds.

The want to address this topic with you emerged following an exchange with the French Bench Press Recordman Baptiste Marchais (also known under the name Bench&Cigars on social media) during which we discussed about the influence the length of anatomical segments for disciplines linked to strength. Following that, I asked myself many questions and I then conducted some research to find answers to these ones. It also occurred to me hearing "theory might well be very nice, but nothing is worth the field". Admittedly. So, my turn to ask questions regarding the arguments "I will never be good in that because of my long segments" without falling into extremes (it would be absurd comparing someone living with dwarfism to Usain Bolt in athletics for example):

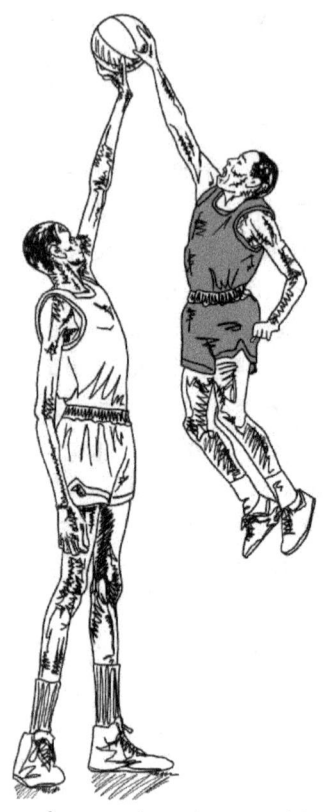

Has this argument prevented Redon Manushi to beat the French record on the snatch (weightlifting) despite his long arms?

Has this argument prevented Muggsy Bogues to become a renown NBA player despite his small height?

Has this argument prevented Julius Maddox to become the Bench Press record man despite his long arms?

Has this argument prevented Nate Robinson to become a multiple champion of Slam Dunk Contest in NBA despite his small height?

If we had directed these athletes towards a "more suitable" discipline from their birth with regards to their anthropometry, we would probably have missed something incredible, don't you think?

There could be other examples to be given, these are not the only ones!

The argument "I will never be good in that because my morpho-anatomy does not allow me to" only takes into account one single factor:

The length of bone segments.

The problem is that other factors are completely overlooked without citing a clear goal, such as:

- Adaptation

- Technique

- Muscle density

- The use of elastic energy...

Don't you see where I want to go despite the explanations related to the aforementioned scientific studies? Let me give you an example:

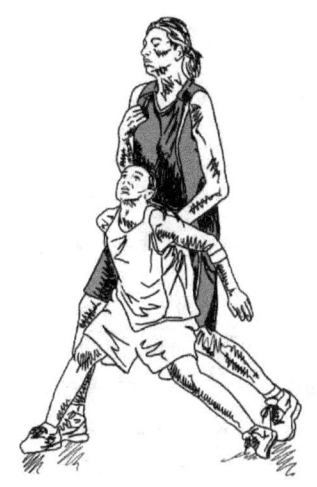

Let's assume that two individuals want to do Bench Press competition.

Individual A measures 1m91 with a scale of 2 metres and a muscle density of 100kg (this is what we call having a big trunk or torso). On the other hand, Individual B measures 1m91 with a scale of 1m96 and a muscle density of 85kg.[31]

---

[31] The examples given are simplified as much as possible to facilitate the understanding of the larger public. Of course, other factors could be included such as structural and nervous factors, notions of specificity related to movement, sporting history...

Put aside external factors (often uncontrollable for a coach in his framework) such as sleep, potential pathologies, nutrition, etc. Let's assume that the two individuals train with the same frequency and with the same goal: performing on a single and unique movement, the Brench Press.

Do you still think that Individual A would lose simply because of the fact that he has longer segments? Probably not. By the way, this has been indicated above.

As a coach or as a training partner, perhaps you have already heard:

"Yes but I don't do competitions. I just want to feel good. In addition, I don't like this movement."

No problem! That is to be respected!

That is why I also mention the adaptation factor. As a coach or as an accompanying person, you must adapt by taking into account the adherence of the individual under supervision. If the individual under supervision considers that their morphology does not allow them to optimise muscle recruitment on a movement which has been programmed, you should know that the movement can be adapted! That might be through an incline, an adaptation of the equipment, ...

Some examples?

The Bench Press, according to him, is not optimal in terms of chest recruitment because of his long arms? The Decline Press can be a solution.

The Front Squat does not allow him to correctly recruit his quadriceps and he leans forward too much or his scapular belt mobility is not optimal? You can test the Zercher Squat which can be very interesting for quadriceps recruitment whilst keeping the back straighter.[32]

In short, there is something for everyone!

As Redon Manushi said:

"In weightlifting, I've always been limited by my physique but I've never wanted to listen to the people who told me that I was maybe not built for that. My relentlessness in my trainings allowed me to maximally optimise my weak physical means. Morphology and physical qualities are important but they are only two factors amongst many others."

Conclusion:

Although we might suppose that anthropometry is important and that it influences sports performance, that one should not hold you back from your progression. It only constitutes one single factor of performance amongst many others. What matters is to find solutions to optimisation and/ or adaptation to levers.

---

[32] Zercher Squat: By the way, I released a youtube video on the "MindFit BXL" channel on this topic which explains you the numerous benefits of that movement.

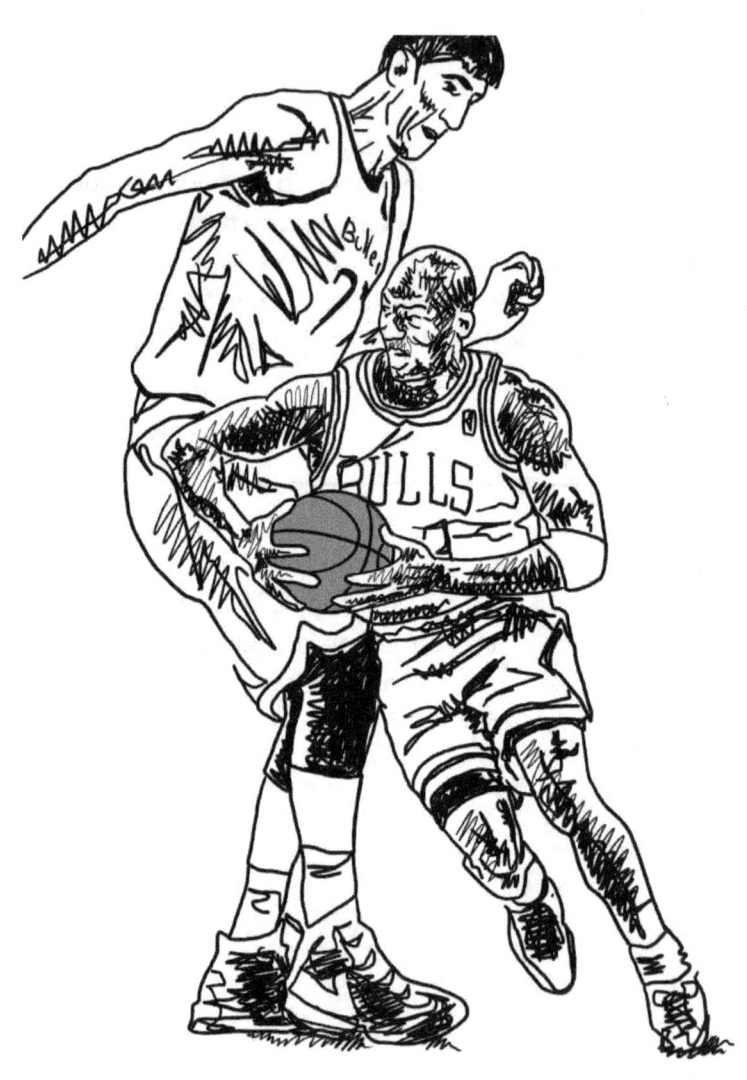

21. I lack stability

I've already said it a few times when I fail an exercise, and I still surprise myself saying it from time to time when I train or when I train a client.

What is stability?

If we refer ourselves to the definition coming from the dictionary, it means:

"Characteristic of what tends to remain in the same state."

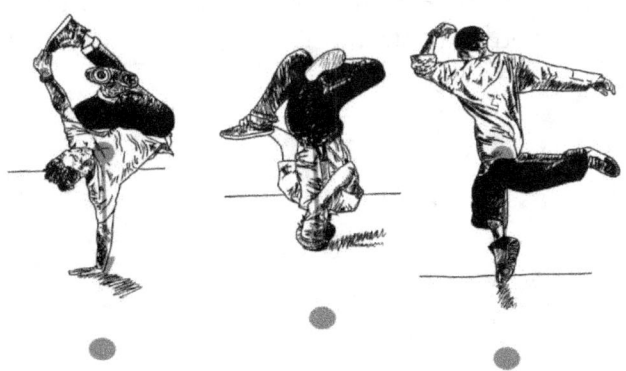

But does the fact of failing a movement come from stability?

Is it a lack of stability which brings failure during a movement?

Well, as said by Olivier Bolliet[33], the concept of stability in of itself, does not exist.

---

[33] Olivier Bolliet is a physical trainer for professional athletes (Olympic Games, World championships and European Championships). He is also co-author of the book "La préparation physique moderne" ("Modern physical preparation") written with Aurélien Broussal-Derval.

If we fail a movement, if we lose balance, it will essentially come from a lack of joint mobility and/ or of strength.

Of course, that is valid at the exception of a potential specific pathology.

> Conclusion:
>
> Failing/ missing a movement is directly correlated to a lack of joint mobility and/ or of strength.

22. Weight training and/ or weightlifting is dangerous and destroys growth (in teens)

It is a belief that still regularly comes up, and yet![xxvii]

We still here:

"It is bad for the joints"

"It prevents from growing taller"

"It destroys growth"

"It is dangerous and of no use!"

Really?

How many times have I not heard these kind of arguments... and yet!

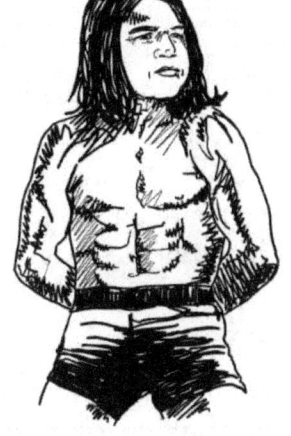

The practice of weight training is defined as an array of physical exercises aimed towards the development of skeletal muscles in order to acquire more strength, endurance, power, explosiveness or muscle density.

Having already lingered on the topic, and particularly on youth development via weightlifting[xxviii], here is what arises as a result:

1)   Not one sport has a negative influence on a child's growth. On the contrary, weightlifting could favour growth: Faigenbaum[xxix] has reported that elite teenager weightlifters who regularly train with heavy loads have a level of bone mineral density way superior than the average, as the muscular forces which act upon the bones to perform the desired movement can be a stimulus for bone formation (osteogenesis).

2) According to many studies, the rate of injury in weightlifting is inferior comparatively to that encountered in other sports (rugby, football, basket, tennis, ...)

Many scientific studies looking at injuries across different sporting disciplines, by the way, allow saying that weightlifting is a safe practice, rarely source of injury. Moreoover, a study published in 1999 by a team of American researchers, conducted on American high-level weightlifters (followed for six years) reveals an injury rate of 3,3 injuries / 1000 hours of training. It is to be noted that the study also took into account competition periods. The down time from training after the noted injuries was mostly inferior to 1 day (for 90,6% of injuries). It therefore appears that injuries in weightlifting are not very severe.

For the sake of comparison, disciplines such as skiing show rates amounting to up to 167 injuries/1000 races. For football, rates of 2,5 to 5,6 injuries/ 1000 hours of training have been shown... And that is, only for hamstring injuries. Even worse, these generated absences from training going well above 1 month! Rates going up to 25,6/1000h in football have been reported. Nonetheless, we often frequently hear people saying "But weightlifting is a dangerous sport".

3) Contrarily to preconceived beliefs, the reinforcement of the back and torso muscles which weightlifting allows prevents injuries and reduces chronic back pain.

4) Concerning growth, it is obvious that in small categories (-56kg, -62 kg for men for example), size is a performance factor. In fact, less dense physiques, meaning taller for a same weight, could not express themselves as they would not dispose of a sufficient muscular support. However, higher

categories allow taller athletes to be able to express themselves. (Dimitry Klokov, 1m83... Does it ring a bell?)

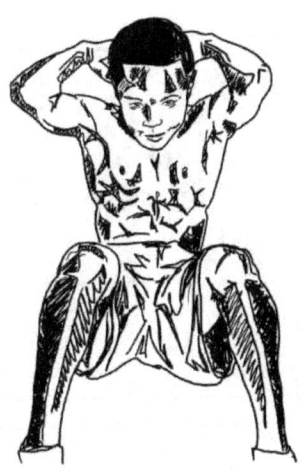

So, in what ways is weightlifting (and weight training) beneficial for children?

- It gets joints working and it strengthens almost all muscles
- A well led learning process constitutes an act of prevention for chronic low back pain (Dr Renault)
- Weightlifting and practising movements with low loads contribute to the general development of children motricity (Renault)
- Weightlifting develops strength, speed, coordination and flexibility
- Weightlifting can be realised as much by men as it can be by women. Rules are adapted depending on the sex (e.g.: weight of the barbell, weight categories, ...)

The most effective period to develop strength and speed qualities starts from mid-puberty. That is when the hormonal situation is at its peak.

> Conclusion:
>
> Weight training and weightlifting do not have negative influences on a child's growth. On the contrary, they bring some benefits (if well supervised).

23. I am too old to gain muscle

Well, we will not lie and give false hopes to the individuals who would like to start and who are above their forties.

However!

Certain people continue to believe that it is too late to develop ourselves muscularly because of hormonal reductions in the body.

Even though it is harder to build muscle passed 25/26 years old, it remains totally possible to develop ourselves muscularly. Admittedly, the more the body ages, the harder recovery is. The more we age, the more the growth potential diminishes.

But as explained in Article 19, if you start weight training, it is totally possible to obtain muscle gains as a novice, and that, even with a low frequency of twice per week. However, reached a certain point, regardless of age, it will be required to increase training frequency to at least three times per week whilst maintaining that regularly if you want to avoid stagnation.

In short, it is still possible!

Conclusion:

Age is just a number, you can progress. There is no age to start weight training.

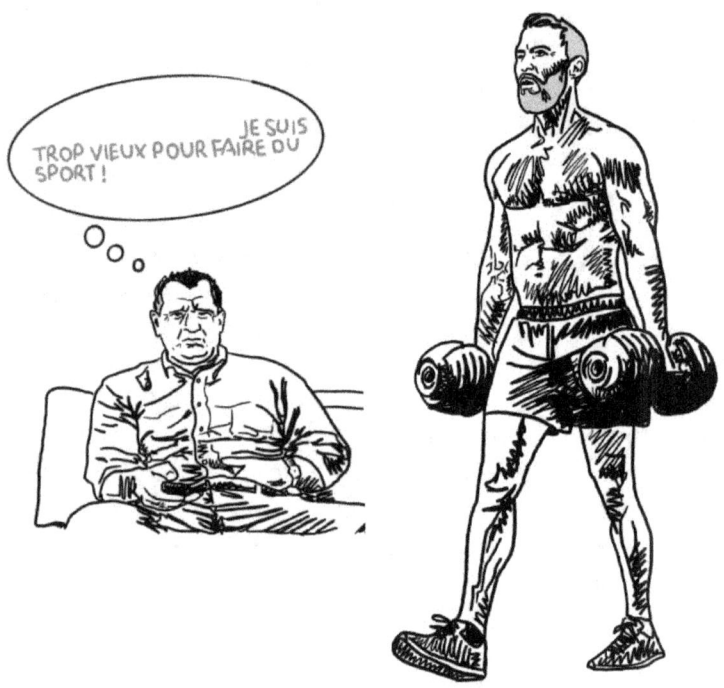

24. CROSSFIT Pull Ups are useless, you might as well do strict Pull Ups

"CrossFit" Pull Ups, also coined Butterfly Pull Ups" (the term Kipping Pull Ups or even Muscle Up exist with the foundations of the movements being similar, but where certain differences are apparent) are often topics of controversy and compared to traditional Pull Ups, more often referred to as "Strict Pull Up".

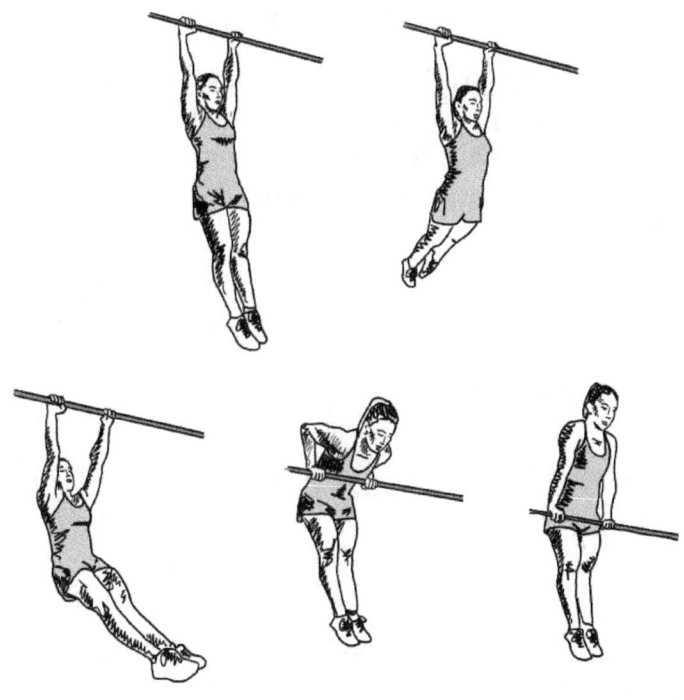

The main difference between a traditional Pull Up (Strict Pull Up – mostly found in Fitness and Bodybuilding circles[34]) is the fact that we will use/ create momentum to reduce the muscular effort to the benefit of elastic and kinetic energy thanks to a deloading of lower limbs. This has the advantage of allowing to do more of them and/ or do them faster.

Why that?

Don't forget CrossFit's initial goal: performing exercises with the purpose of acquiring the physical condition allowing to work at a certain intensity rate (sometimes with a high training volume) but also gestural techniques to reduce energy consumption to not exhaust yourself in 30 seconds, and ending unable to pursue the work to be done.

Thereby, thanks to these techniques, you reduce your dependency on torso muscles (necessary force). Yet, you accentuate your dependence to the mobility of 2 chains (scapular and hip), as well as to your coordination level (Top/ bottom).

In short, here are the effects of "Butterfly Pull Ups":

- Work on coordination
- Work on the spine's elasticity
- Work on flexibility
- Work on the mobility of the scapular and hip chains
- Work on explosiveness
- Work on physical condition (endurance)
- Work on speed

As a reminder, CrossFit and bodybuilding are 2 different and not comparable disciplines.

---

[34] We also find Strict Pull Ups in the disciplines of street workout like the set&reps or in street lifting

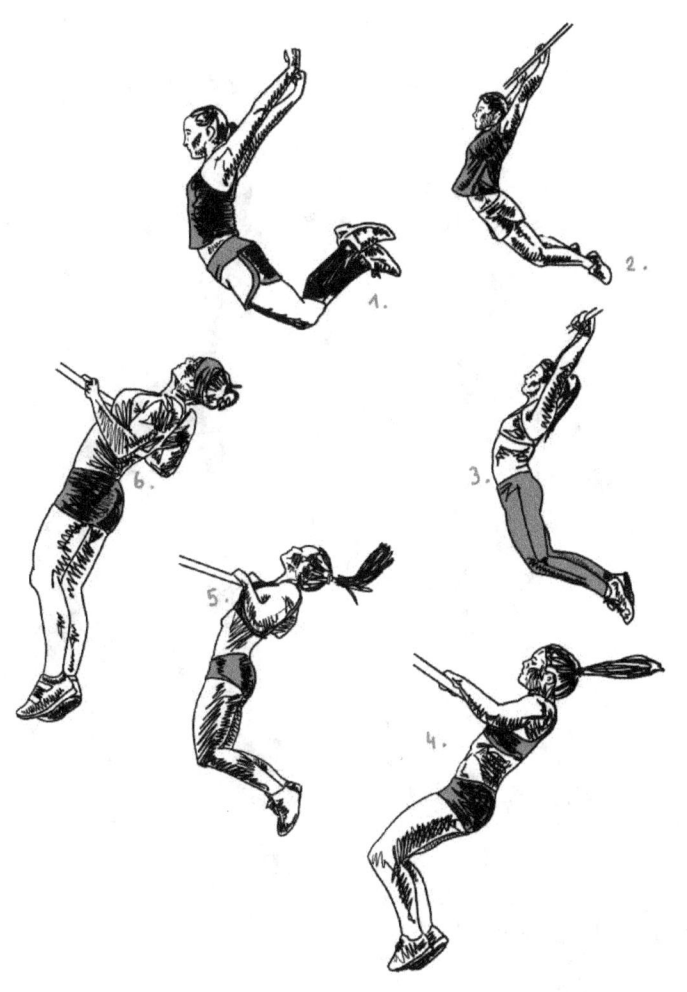

Conclusion:

Pull Ups which we see in the CrossFit space are not useless. It really depends on the goal.

25. The goal is not to be strong in one area, but to be strong everywhere

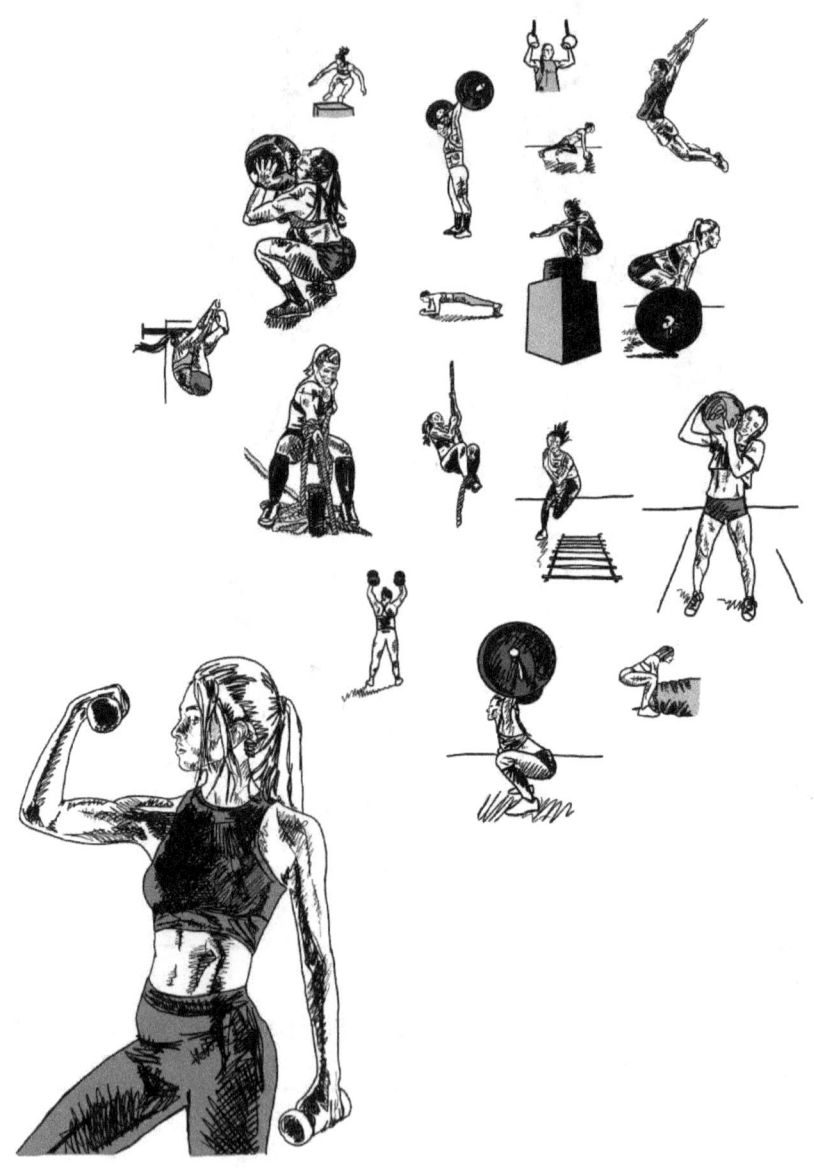

That is, without the shadow of a doubt, the sentence I see the most on social media when it comes to CrossFit!

Mmmmh how to put it?

The best way to counterbalance that saying is to state a quote which sticks in my mind since I've heard it:

"The goal of CrossFit is not to be strong everywhere but to fail nowhere"

This already gets us back on the right track. Well, now that we have made things clear, how can we explain that?

We know it, CrossFit is a mix between different disciplines:

- Weightlifting
- Gymnastics
- Kettlebell sport/Girevoy Sport
- Powerlifting
- Endurance sports

Knowing that CrossFit positions itself around several athletic competencies: muscular and respiratory endurance, strength, flexibility, power, speed, agility, psychomotor skills, balance and precisions.

Although exceptions such as the athlete Tia-Clair Toomey[35] exist, do you think it is fundamentally possible to perform at a high level in as many domains?

---

[35] Tia-Clair Toomey is 5x champion of the CrossFit Games. She also participated to the 2016 Olympic Games in weightlifting where she obtained the 14th place.

A word of caution, the goal is not to criticise CrossFit. Far from that. Clearly, CrossFit allowed to put forward certain disciplines which were unknown from the general public (e.g. weightlifting and kettlebell sport/girevoy sport). However, being strong everywhere is impossible because you must sometimes fully dedicate a part of your life to attain an exemplary level.

Rather than thinking that the goal of CrossFit is to be strong everywhere, I think it would be preferable to think that the strength of CrossFit lies in its versatility.

<u>To be taken into account:</u>

CrossFit has been "run down" in every possible way regarding its ability to mix strength and cardiovascular training forms which could lead to "concurrent zones" in training. Although opinions vary a lot between coaches as it relates to the fact of mixing (or not) cardio and weight training in a single session, it is important not to generalise.

The first thing that should not be mixed up are the goals of the disciplines relating to concurrent zones. This principally relates to hypertrophy. Which is, to my knowledge, the first goal of a CrossFit athlete. Then, according to different studies[xxx], it would appear that the reduction of glycogen stores (energy substrates) and that residual fatigue could potentially be the cause of decreased performances, and so, of muscle gains. That means that adding cardio when the goal is hypertrophy for which volume remains a centrepiece could strongly negatively impact the hypertrophy work.

Therefore, the nuance to add is that the accumulation of working volume and goal prioritisation, rather than cardio activity in of itself, is what appears to be problematic regarding muscle gains. In addition, a form of cardio is necessary for performance and for health (longevity). Consequently, it is important to include some cardio in your training programme, but by taking into account energy and fatigue management.

> Conclusion:
>
> CrossFit's strength comes from its technical versatility. It is also important to memorise that a concurrent zone between hypertrophy and cardio within a session does exist, but that this one does not necessarily mean that cardiovascular work harms hypertrophy as long as the level of priority of the goal as well the energy levels are respected.

26. Do not do CrossFit, you will injure yourself!

It is funny how this sentence comes back regularly, and it is even said by certain doctors and sometimes even by sedentary individuals who have never tried CrossFit!

So... is it true?

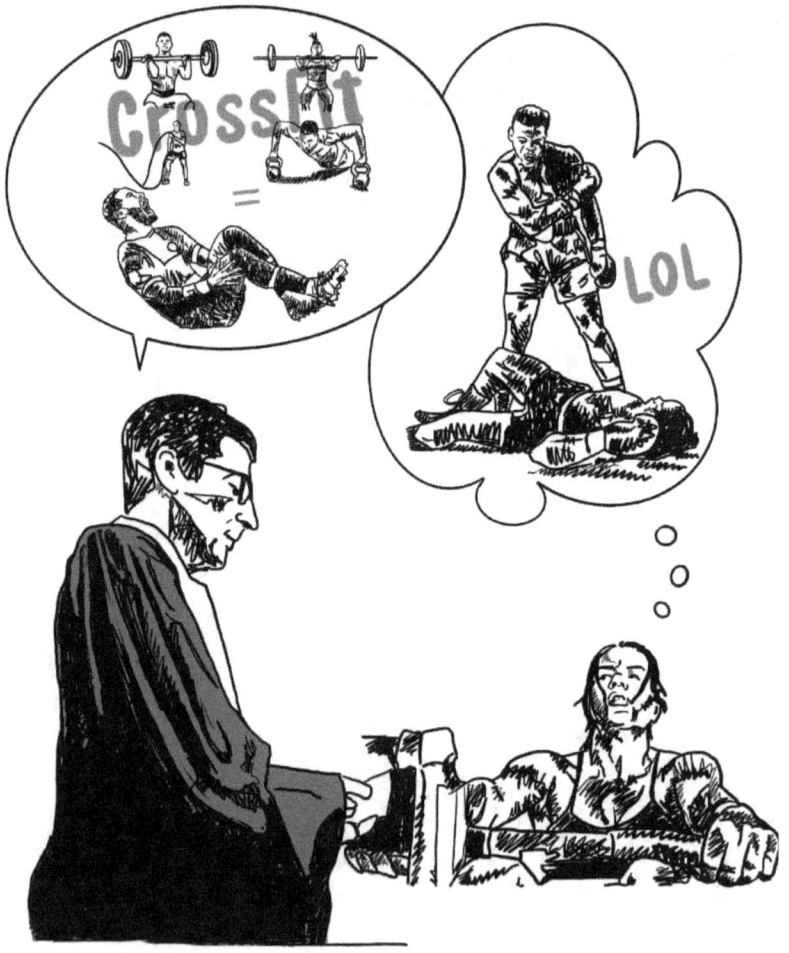

From an external viewpoint, we could understand why CrossFit might frighten as it can make us step out from habits that we are used to seeing in weight training.

And obviously, when we are not accustomed to something and when it steps outside the norm, we could think that it is dangerous as we are seeing movements with large ranges of motion, the lifting of impressive loads, etc.

A study issued in 2013[xxxi] explained that out of 97 participants, 73,5% underwent an injury which prevented them to pursue their physical activity or even working. Even worse. 7% had to undergo a surgical intervention.

If we stop there, these numbers are clearly worrying.

However, it is important to put things into perspective. An injury rate of 3.1 for 1000 hours of training has been calculated to allow a comparison with other sports.

The injury rate for 1000 hours of training would be similar to that of strength sports such as weightlifting or powerlifting, or that of fitness, and even that of running.

The most recurring injuries were found on the shoulders and on the lower back.

BUT!

The authors have admitted that this study suffers from several limitations. Firstly, the low number of participants does not allow for a real comparison with the injury rate calculated in other disciplines on a much broader public. The fact of proposing a questionnaire on injuries could have encouraged individuals who injured themselves to participate to it. In addition, the answers did not specify under which circumstances the injuries arose.

Clearly, CrossFit is not more dangerous than weight training in the gym, gymnastics or running. All the more so, you are supervised by a coach during a session in a CrossFit box. That is not always the case in weight training.

A few more recent studies which came out in 2017[xxii] and in 2018[xxiii] have demonstrated that CrossFit did not give rise to more risks than another physical intensity performed at high intensity thresholds.

Conclusion:

CrossFit is not more dangerous than weight training in a gym, gymnastics or even running.

27. I will lose all my gains if I do not train during a week

No panic! Although fitness is sometimes considered to be an ungrateful sport (we have all already heard "as soon as you stop, you will lose everything"), it is important to take a step back.

Be it fitness or whatever other physical activity, as you stop practising during a certain period of time, it is difficult to return to what was once your level right from the start. But thankfully, there is muscle memory.

Muscle memory, what is it?

Muscle memory is a form of procedural memory which consists of consolidating a specific memorised motor task under the effect of repetition, which has been used synonymously with motor learning.[xxiv]

To understand what muscle memory really was and the impact that this one had on the body, a study[xxv] published in 2016 asked to 23 sedentary participants to train only one of their two legs during a defined timeframe (a bit below an hour). The exercise has been repeated four times per week on a period equivalent to one trimester. Then, after a long downtime, the study's participants went back to training but they now worked both their legs.

The team conducted biopsies[36] before and after the exercise

---

[36] Sampling a tissue fragment on a living being in sight of a microscopic test ("Le Robert" French Dictionary)

periods to see which genes were active. The results show that gene expression was similar in both legs, despite only one leg having been trained for three months.

But then? Does muscle memory really exist?

Although the results of this study suggest that muscles do not keep the exercise in memory, the situation is different concerning nerve cells which control movement. The nerve system learns in which order activate muscles to execute a movement (for example: riding a bicycle, putting a foot in front of the other to walk, catching a ball, driving a car, ...)

"Yes, but you are going astray! I just want to know how long it will take for me to lose my gains."

I'm getting there!

Now that we have explained what muscle memory is, and that even if you experience some muscle loss due to a long period of inactivity, you have the possibility to get back to your previous level (with the exception of serious pathologies which occurred in the meantime or other specific cases).

How much time before a loss of muscle mass?

A 2017 study revealed that when trained individuals take two weeks off from strength-related training, muscle size does not diminish to a significant degree[xxxvi]

Another research review goes a bit further and suggests that taking up to 3 weeks off from training does not significantly influence the size of muscles[xxxvii]

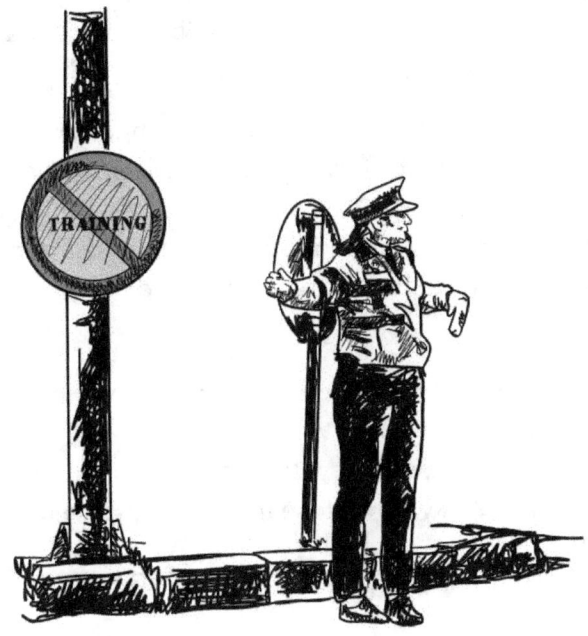

"Yes, maybe, but I still have the impression of losing weight after so many days off from training"

Indeed, that is an impression that certain individuals have already shared with me… But to what could this be due?

We suggest[37] that the reason why we tend to feel "skinnier/thinner" after an absence of training of a few days to a few weeks would be linked to a reduction of muscle glycogen stores, making muscles "a little bit smaller"[xxxviii].

---

37   Hypothesis*

However, looking at the real size of muscles, the latter can be maintained during many weeks without training.

In a research review[xxxix], it has been noticed that with only 1 to 2 training sessions per week, it is possible to maintain your muscles for at least 32 weeks.

For individuals who travel a lot and who cannot access a gym during a certain period of time (due to decisions linked to a pandemic for example), Bill Campbell[38][xl] suggests resistance training by getting close to muscular failure to maintain our level, or even, to certain extents, continue to progress.

Conclusion:

There is no reason to worry if you miss one, two, three or seven days of training. You will not lose muscle mass, even after two weeks off.

---

[38] Bill Campbell is a professor of motricity sciences and a scientist. He is also the director of the laboratory "Performance&Physique Enhancement"

28. The deadlift, the king of exercises, essential in bodybuilding

I feel like we are going to spit on me! Let's calm down. At least, wait until I provide you with certain explanations.

I have a keen interest in powerlifting and in strength-related sports more generally. It is a discussion I had with a powerlifter which made me want to write this article. At one point, that athlete told me:

"If you don't do powerlifting, weightlifting or CrossFit, the Deadlift is useless apart for injuring yourself ("finir flingué" in French)[39]!"

Well, I admit that it is difficult to hear. Difficult, certainly, but it maybe not that unreasonable. Let me explain myself:

We could rather say that the Deadlift is of "almost no use". As mentioned above, it has its purpose in CrossFit, in weightlifting and in powerlifting.

As such, should we ban the Deadlift of our training? NO!

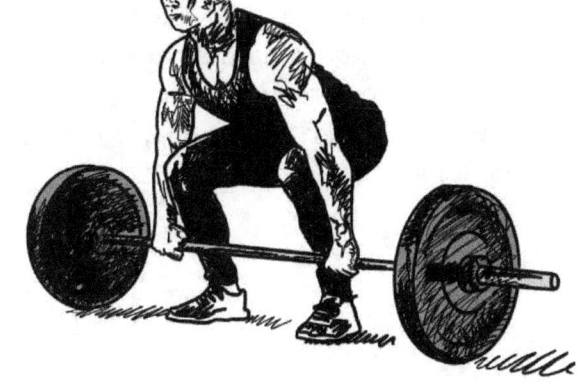

---

[39] "Finir flingué" is a French expression which means "injuring yourself" in that context.

However, some alternatives which would be more interesting for other sporting disciplines do exist.

For example, in the case of hypertrophy/ muscle growth, a Romanian Deadlift will be more interesting since it will involve a larger range of motion and more tension on the posterior chain. In addition, the injury risk will be reduced as compared to a conventional Deadlift because the load will be lighter as a result of its execution.

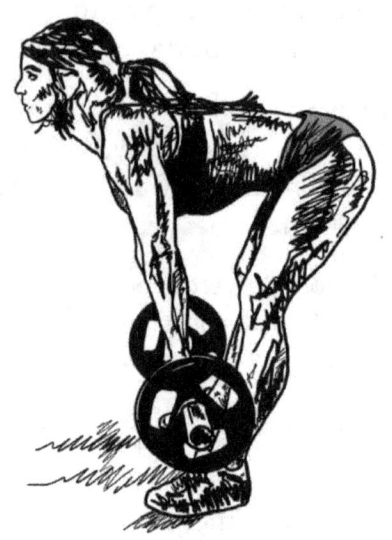

Another example would also be to perform a Deadlift but with a trap/Hex barbell rather than with an Olympic Barbell. A study showed that bringing the barbell closer to the vertical axis of the body allows reducing mechanical constraints applied on the lower back and on the hip, which could potentially allow reducing traumas.

That difference in terms of positioning also allows generating a speed and a power significantly superior to that of traditional/conventional Deadlift.[xli]

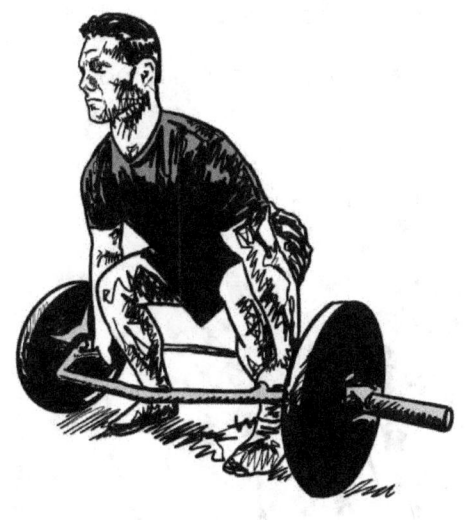

It is recommended to keep the "traditional Deadlift" as a priority exercise for strength athletes or for athletes which encounter some Deadlift in their discipline. In case of the contrary, all athletes which are not strength specialists would derive more benefit from using an alternative to the conventional Deadlift. They would obtain more advantages from those.

Conclusion:

Depending on the context, the conventional Deadlift is not essential.

29. Heyyy Patriciiiia! Guess what!? I've bought a new trendy cream which just got out to make cellulite disappear!

Well, I'll give you that, the title is seducing!

It is true that it is a problem that most women have due to the simple reason that it is neither "beautiful" nor "aesthetic".

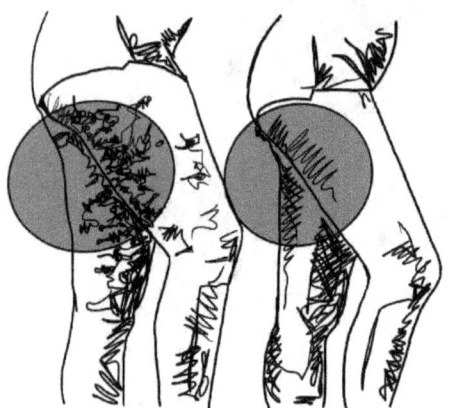

That topic has already been covered by a large number of health and sports professionals, but it is a perduring myth, so I must add my contribution!

The first thing to know is that cellulite does not result from holding too high of a bodyfat percentage. So, do not damage your health by trying to slim down too rapidly in the hope of losing some cellulite. It is dangerous and useless.

Nonetheless, it is true that bodyfat can aggravate the situation when we have cellulite. It is to be noted that cellulite concerns most women. These women could be slim, overweight, with blonde hair, with brown or with red hair, might they get up at the crack of dawn or not! You've got it, you are not the only one (woman but also man) to have cellulite. It is common and it would even concern above 85% of women! (For men, I would not be able to tell you!)

The second myth regards the treatment of cellulite.

As of today, there is no effective treatment allowing to definitely make cellulite disappear. You will effectively have short term results, but on the long term, no product could guarantee you to completely make cellulite disappear (apart from false advertisings of course… "Well well well"!)

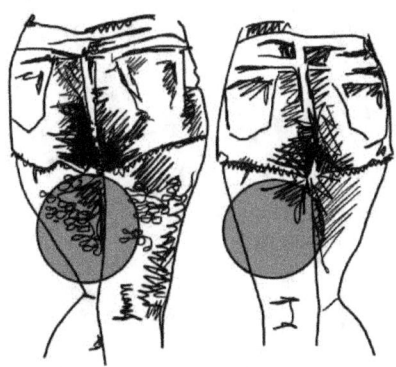

Several studies[xlii] have confirmed those words by taking into account the different possible types of treatments such anti-cellulite creams, massages, infrared treatments, …

In brief, the best you can do is to exercise and to learn how to "eat better". This will allow reducing your bodyfat percentage and getting a nicer silhouette. Put simply, you will be "more aesthetic"!

Conclusion:

No treatment will allow to completely make cellulite disappear. Having cellulite is natural.

30. <u>If I weigh as much, it is because I have big bones.</u>

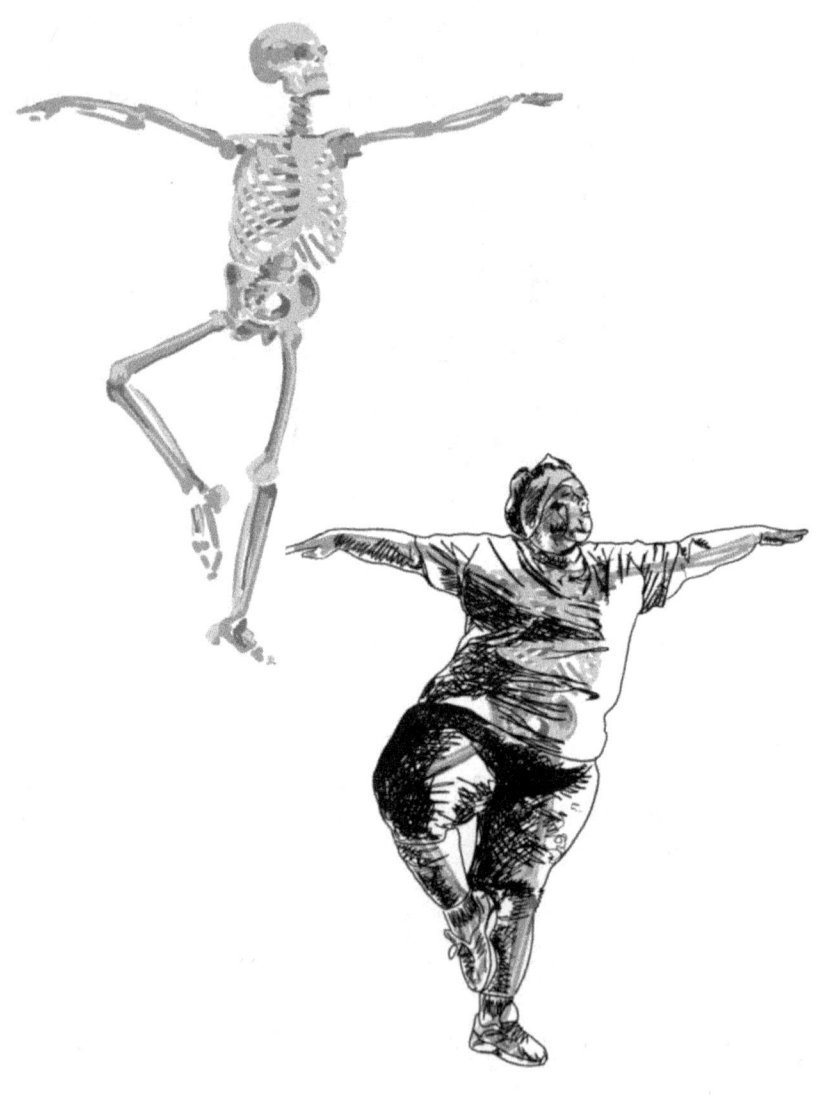

To give you an explanation of why this is absurd, the best to do is to collect data from reliable sources.

El Sabre[40] had published an article which very well summarised that heavy bones do not explain an excess of weight. These words have by the way also been said by Bengt Kayser, Professor at the "Institut de la médecine du sport - Université de Genève" (Institute of Sports Medecine – Geneva University).

The explanations are very clear:

"In humans, bones only represent about 15% of total body weight, and a difference between density and bone volume will only have a low impact on total weight.

What makes body weight change the most is muscular volume (think of a bodybuilder) or bodyfat volume (think of obesity); in both cases, we can accumulate a dozen of kilos.

Heavy bones are therefore not an explanation for an excess of weight."

Conclusion:

Heavy bones are not the explanation behind being overweight.

---

[40] El Sabre is renowned on social media where he covers different topics, techniques, ideas and training equipment.

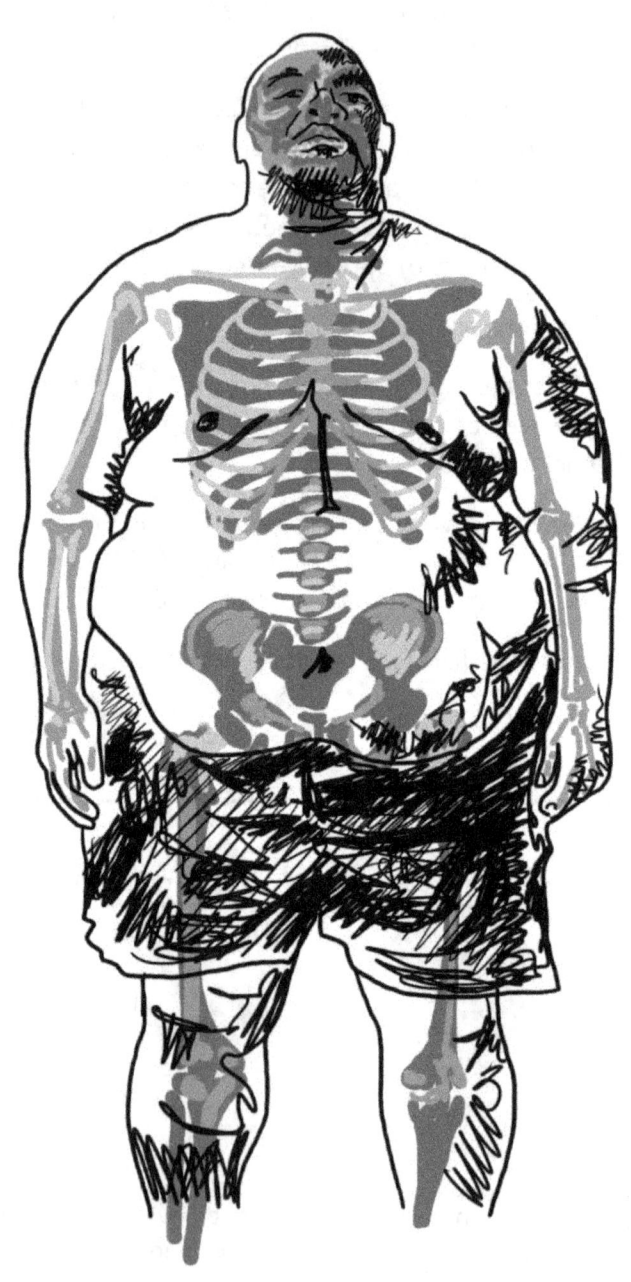

31. The squat recruits as much of the leg muscles possible, you cannot find more complete!

I agree on the fact that the squat is a complete exercise. It is quite simple, if I had to select a single exercise amongst all those which exist, I would choose the squat (with an analysis of the goal and of the adherence of the individual in charge of course).

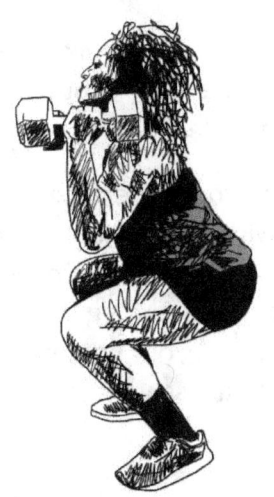

However, the fact that squat would recruit as much of the leg muscles as possible… not sure about that! In all case, not to their maximum.

Chris Beardsley[41], shared an analysis from the journal "Strength & Conditioning research"[xiii] effectively demonstrating that the squat worked the leg muscles well, but to a completely level recruitment rate!

The study compared three types of squats. The Back Squat with complete range of motion (full squat), the Front Squat and the Parallel Squat which corresponds to a squat a little bit below the 90 degrees angle.

---

[41] Chris Beardsley is a scientist specialised in sports research

For all variations used, quadriceps activation was high, BUT hamstring activation was relatively low.

It is to be noted that it is not specified whether the squat was High Bar (above the trapezius muscles) or Low Bar (below the trapezius muscles). We are presuming it was high bar.

It also seems like the squat does not optimally develop the rectus femori muscle, one of the four heads of the quadriceps muscle.[xliv]

It would therefore be recommended to associate the squat with hip flexion exercises (e.g. Romanian Deadlift), but also with knee genuflection and extension exercises (e.g. Leg Curl as well as Leg Extension[xlv] or Reverse Nordic Curl) to best recruit your posterior chain and your rectus femoris in order to maximise your muscle gains on your legs.

Conclusion:

Variations in the depth of the Back Squat or squat variations do not possess an elevated muscle activation threshold for the hamstrings and the rectus femoris. It is therefore important to supplement the squat with other exercises to maximum gains on the legs.

32. The Deadlift is more tiring than the Squat!

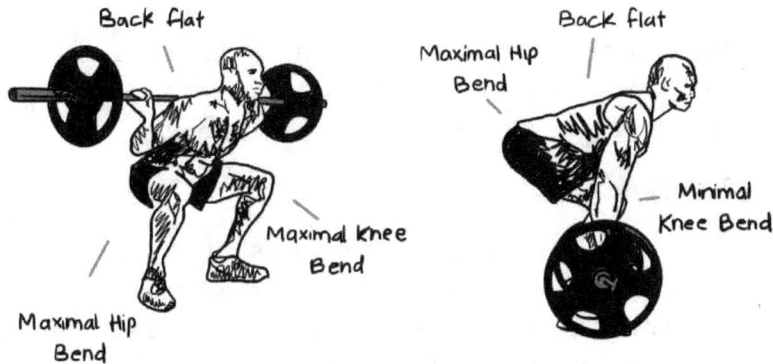

Here is a topic which comes out a lot between science enthusiasts and those of the field! Although everyone is different and that some may have more ease on one exercise rather than on another depending on various factors, what does the science say regarding the comparison of the Deadlift (conventional Deadlift) and of the squat (Back Squat) in terms of fatigue?

Central fatigue[42][xlvi] and peripheral fatigue[43] are the backbones which make most of the differences.

---

[42] Central fatigue occurs in the CNS (central nervous system). It includes all the mechanisms which alter the generation of the motor command and the recruitment of motor units, both on the spinal and on the supraspinal levels (brain and spinal cord).

[43] Peripheral fatigue corresponds to disturbances to the muscle's capacity to produce force. Nevertheless, experimental observations show that a peripheral modification acts on a central level on the recruitment of motor units. Muscular damage and metabolic stress in your muscles are an example of peripheral fatigue. Their effects are local and specific to the muscle in which they occur.

In fact, a study[xlvii] demonstrated that fatigue on the Deadlift was overall similar to that on the squat.

Nonetheless, a slight difference with peripheral fatigue is noted as it is more important on the squat movement. That is probably due to a bigger work done by the quadriceps.

<u>To be taken into account:</u>

Regarding powerlifting competitors, it would seem that peaking (the process aimed at maximising the preparation for a given moment) tends to show that there is a need for a little bit more rest on the deadlift before a competition.

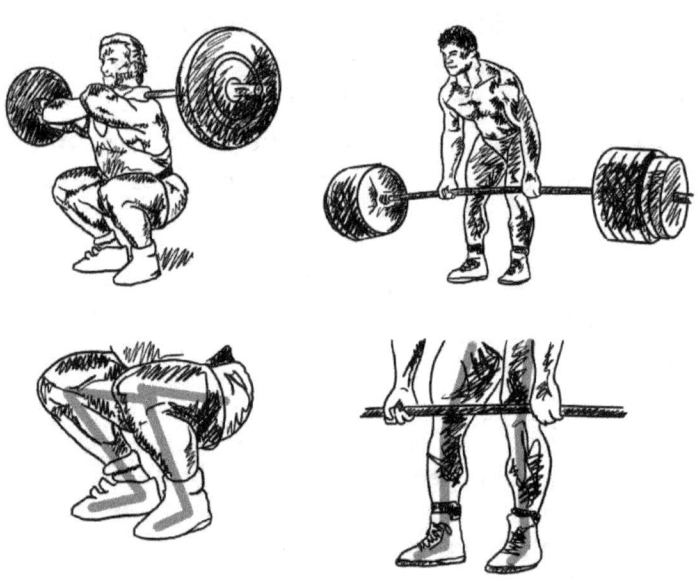

Conclusion:

Apart for powerlifting competitors during a peaking where it is suggested to pay attention to the athlete's state, the deadlift is not more tiring than the squat.

33. A woman must not train like a man

As a coach, I've heard this idea on many occasions at the gym. It is false![xlviii]

Of course, at the exception of certain specific cases (e.g. pregnant woman or menstruating woman) for which training will be adapted to the specificity at hand, all type of training can suit for one or for the other.

The goals are what will differ regarding training. Hence the importance of individualising a training programme.

There are nonetheless genetic and physiological differences to take into account between women and men. In fact, it has been proven[xlix] that women have a quadriceps[44] predominance.

This means that it can be interesting to wisely integrate isolation exercises and to encourage the adaptability of the individual without falling into the trap of a nocebo[45] discourse concerning potential instabilities.[46] Asymmetries are normal[l] and they are not problematic for the practise of sports as long as the training is realised progressively.

---

[44] The research proving that women are quadriceps dominant is to be taken with a step back. This only represents one single research, and above all, in specific conditions with the analysis of a single movement. Other studies are to be realised to support the idea, but this remains an interesting indication.

[45] We speak of a nocebo effect when either the psychological or the physiological effect is associated with taking an inert substance leads to detrimental effects for the individual.

[46] An asymmetry is not associated with an increased injury risk. One of the rare cases to take into account is in the case of pain, for which seeking out for support is thus recommended.

And on the level of hypertrophy then?

Studies seem to indicate almost identical results concerning relative gains between men and women. This is quite surprising since we tend to continuously hear that hypertrophy is directly linked to hormones. That does not turn out to be the case. At least, not only. The studies stated here are done mostly on individuals new to weight training. Apparently, demands related to competition seem different (between a male pro bodybuilder and a female pro bodybuilder). In effect, men start with superior muscles masses at a higher level.

Nonetheless, it is important not get mixed up by the fact that, in absolute, men carry more muscle mass than women. That is different from relative gains between both sexes[li].

A woman can therefore follow the programme of a man like a man can follow the programme of a woman. What matters is to ensure that the programme matches the goals of the individual as well as other variables such as sleep and diet (and others still).

Conclusion:

There isn't such a thing as specific exercises for women or for men. It is a question of individualisation.

34. My knees are painful... Certainly due to arthtritis

It is a topic that I have already mentioned with osteopaths, manual therapy trainers and physios! By the way, that debate still comes up regularly. But before making things clear, we must know what arthritis is.

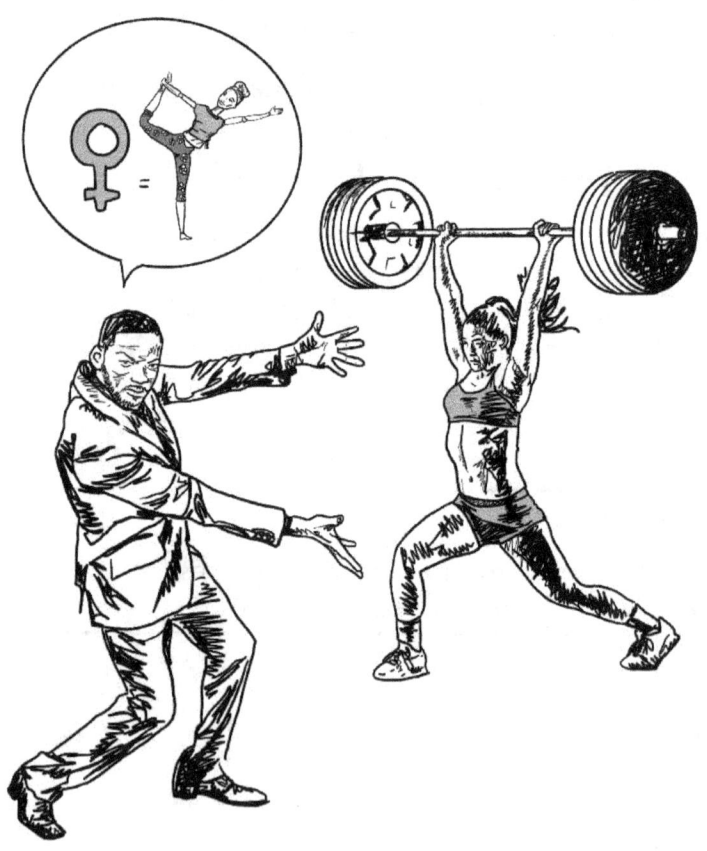

Arthritis is defined as a chronic joint affection due to the deterioration of cartilage[iii]. To put it simply (because let's not kid ourselves, the dictionary's definition is not easy to understand), it is a "thinning" of joint cartilage due to genetic and inflammatory factors.

Having enquired myself with osteopath and physiotherapist friends of mine, they are clear:

There are few links between arthritis and pain (like there sometimes is no correlation between imageries and pain).

> "So then, why do I feel pain?"

Pain can come from many factors such as:

- A lack of Vitamin D

- Anxiety (stress)

- Chronic pain (chronic pains can be improved and reversed)[iiii]

How to mitigate pain?

- By supplementing in Vitamin D if necessary (deficiency)

- By exercising

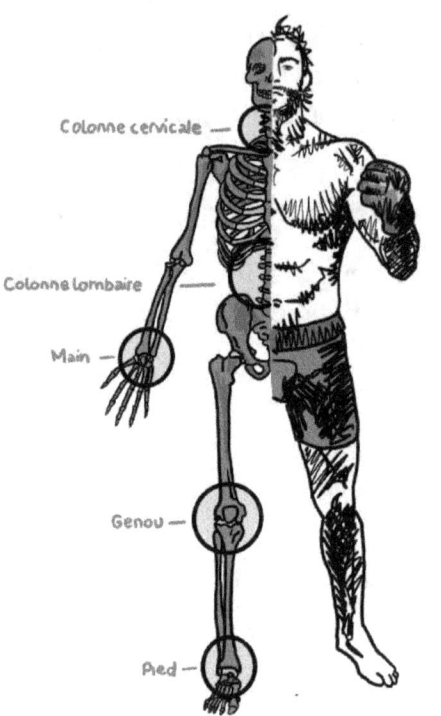

Arthritis is a totally normal phenomenon for an individual. It is not an anomaly and it is a part of life.

Conclusion:

There are very little links between arthritis and pain. Arthritis is not an anomaly and it is a normal life phenomenon.

35. No pain No gain

In Belgium, country of the fry ("la frite" in French) and of the snack where it is possible to stuff yourself for less than 5 euros, we would rather have the tendency to say "No pain, no mitraillette!" (the mitraillette being a Belgian meat sandwich).

Well, now that my terrible joke has been made (and if you didn't understand it, I invite you to order a mitraillette in any snack shop on the Belgian territory), let's directly get back to the fitness world!

The famous "No pain no gain".

A concept which is a little "badass[47]", but also stupid, let me explain:

Firstly, you must know that it is not logical to feel pains during your training when you perform an exercise. I am really speaking of pain here, not of a burning sensation.

Secondly, the fact that you have muscle soreness after your training does not necessarily mean that you worked well.

Do you want a proof? When you are in a feverish state, you can be subject to muscle soreness. And that, having done some sport or not.

Muscle soreness arises when we haven't practiced an exercise or a physical activity since a long time, when we are (sometimes) in a flu-like state, etc.

---

[47] Badass: someone qualified like being "tough"

Concerning muscle soreness, the muscular pain is mostly caused by the body's inflammatory response.[liv]

What should be remembered is that the "No pain No gain" principle is a motivational factor meaning that it is required to work hard and to be disciplined to attain your goals, but that in no cases, you must go to a level of pain during your training, or even after, in the hope of obtaining significant results. If such was the case, we should rename this motivational factor "no Brain no Gain".

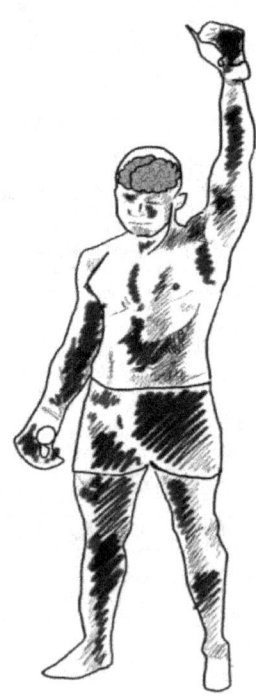

> Conclusion:
>
> You can improve your sports performances as well as your physique/ aesthetics without there being a correlation with muscular pain.

36. Running is dangerous for the knees and for the lower back

In reality, it is the complete opposite! At least, when it is done in a moderate and controlled way.

The popular belief holds that it is dangerous for the back and for the knees because it is a sport with "impacts".

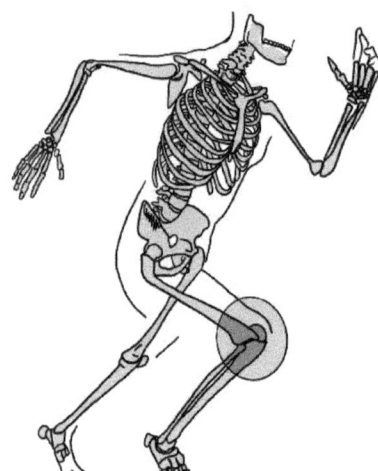

Science has not only showed that there are no correlations between knee arthritis and long distance running[lv], but it has also proven that not going over 30 minutes of running would allow to reduce knee inflammation.[lvi]

And what about back pain?[48]

Practising running on a regular basis would have a positive impact on the back by reinforcing intervertebral discs.[lvii]

---

[48] I had already explained in one of the videos on my youtube channel "Kettlebell Sport: Dangerous for the back?" ("Kettlebell Sport : Dangereux pour le dos ?" in French) by making the connection between running and Kettlebell Sport by looking back at a study published in 2017.

A word of caution though, I want to warn against certain individuals who would want to rush and run never-ending kilometres after having read this book by going back to a sentence coming from my physio which stuck in my mind:

"If there is an injury, it is because we wanted to do too much, too fast. After having done too little for too long, progressivity is the key."

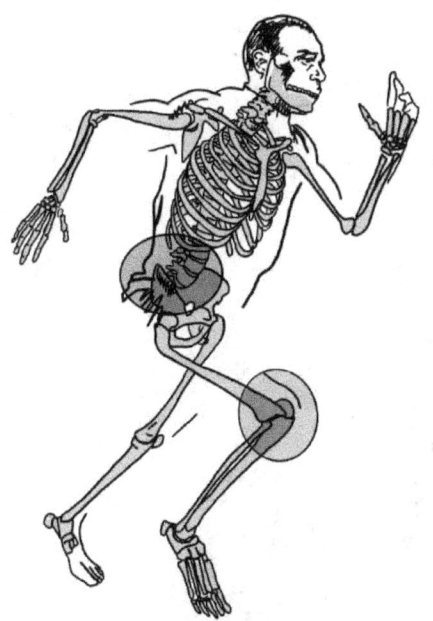

Go for it progressively and enjoy yourself!

Conclusion:
Nor is running dangerous for the knees, nor is it for the back. On the contrary, it can bring certain advantages for these ones.

37. We need to go "harder" on trainings coach, I am not losing weight! There is nothing changing on the scale!

I think that every coach has already heard this idea it at least once. Even more so when we're talking of a beginner who decided to change by seeking the support of a coach.

The fact that you are not seeing your weight go down on the scale does not mean that you are not progressing.

In fact, you must know that as you build muscle, it is possible to lose a certain quantity of fat mass, and to build the same quantity of muscle mass in the same instance. [lviii]

MYTH   Fat takes up 5x more space than muscle
TRUTH   Fat takes up 15% more space than muscle

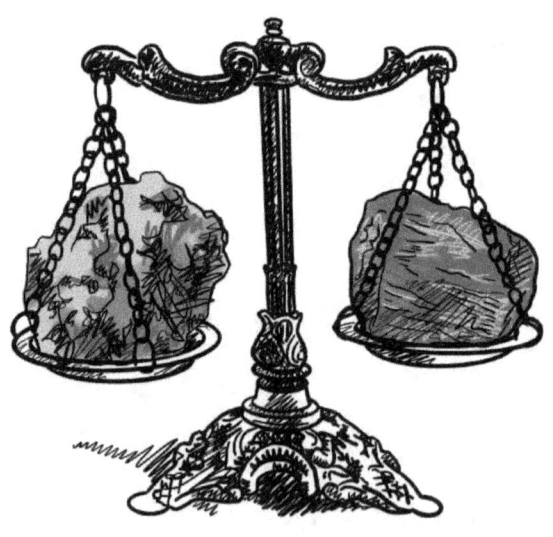

Other thing to take into account: fat tissue takes about 15% more space than muscle. By the way, let's bust a second myth in this article right now, appreciate that fat does not transform into muscle neither. It is burned by the body.

Apart from the scale, here are things you should also pay attention to in order to review your progress:

- The holes in your belt (an additional hole is a sign of progression)
- Mirror (Look at yourself and analyse the change by being proud of yourself)
- The clothes that you were not able to wear anymore (if you still have some, try them on again)
- Your strength is increasing training after training
- You are feeling less tired than previously (improved "energy")

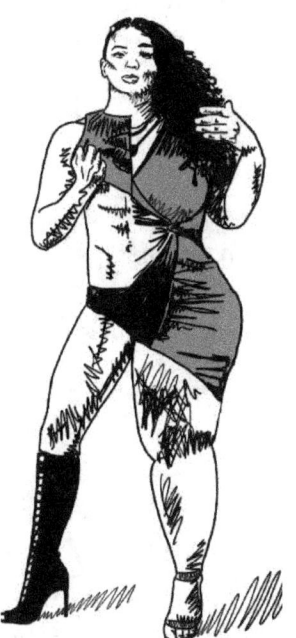

It is to be taken into account that your weight on the scale can change depending on stress, hydration or dehydration, sleep, menstruations (for women), …

Conclusion:

The fact that you are not seeing changes on the scale does not necessarily mean that you are not progressing.

38. Heyyyy Jocelyne? Guess what! I invested in my home gym to lose weight! I bought an elliptical bike, and on my first session I've burned 500 calories using it!

How to be sure that we are really talking of 500 calories? That is precisely the concern!

The following data will influence the number of calories that you can burn during an effort:

- Sex

- Body weight

- General physical condition

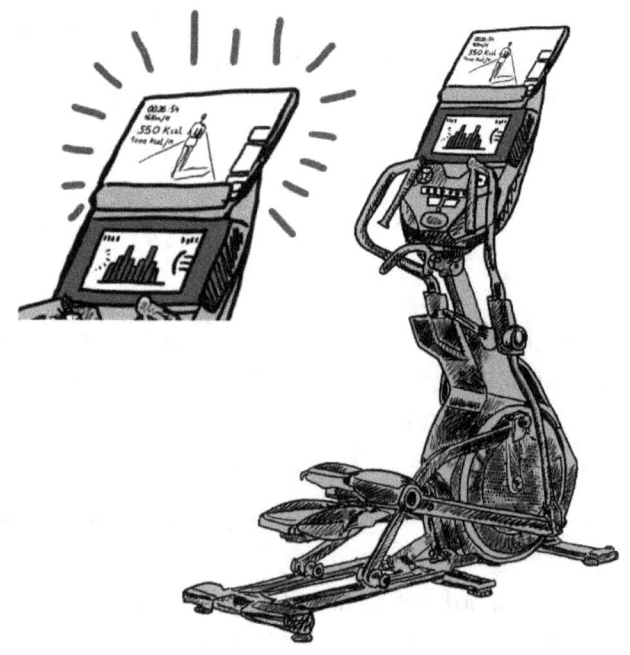

Yet, a machine cannot be reliable because it is not able to take into account all the physiological analyses required. Perhaps this will happen one day with the invasion of artificial intelligence, but in the meantime that is not the case!

In 2010, a study was conduted by the "Human Performance Center"[lix] and the numbers are quite astounding:

- A stationary bike overestimates calorie expenditure by 7%

- A stair climber overestimates energy expenditure by 12%

- A treadmill overestimates energy expenditure by 13%

- An elliptical bike overestimates calorie expenditure by 42%

Roughly speaking, cardio machines tend to overestimate calories burned during an exercise and they do not pay attention to your physiology.

Conclusion:

Think critically regarding the numbers displayed on the counter when you perform your training on a cardio machine.

39. I do cardio before my training session and then I do a big weight training session to cut and build muscle at the same time

It is stupid and it is not difficult to understand.

The unique goal of weight training is to build muscle (logical). By performing a cardio session, you will fatigue yourself physically and nervously. That means that you will not be "fresh" to start your weight training session and that your performances will not be optimal.

What does that mean in terms of consequences?

This comes with the risk of negatively influencing muscle growth.

The advice I would want to give you is to do your cardio at a different moment from your weight training session (example: during an active rest day, excluding any specific goal). In no instance should it be done before your weight/ Fitness training session.

If you lack time during your day or that you are limited by a weekly training frequency, here are the different piece of advice I would give you if your aim is to build muscle mass:

- Favour weight training prior to cardio
- Use an appropriate training method (Full Body, Half-Body, …) depending on your frequency
- Use adequate strategies depending on the time you spend at the gym (e.g. cluster method, training circuits, méthode Legeard, Tabata method, …) without losing sight of your goal.

Conclusion:

Doing a cardio session just before a weight training session will not allow you to have significant gains and it puts you at risk of unnecessarily tiring you.

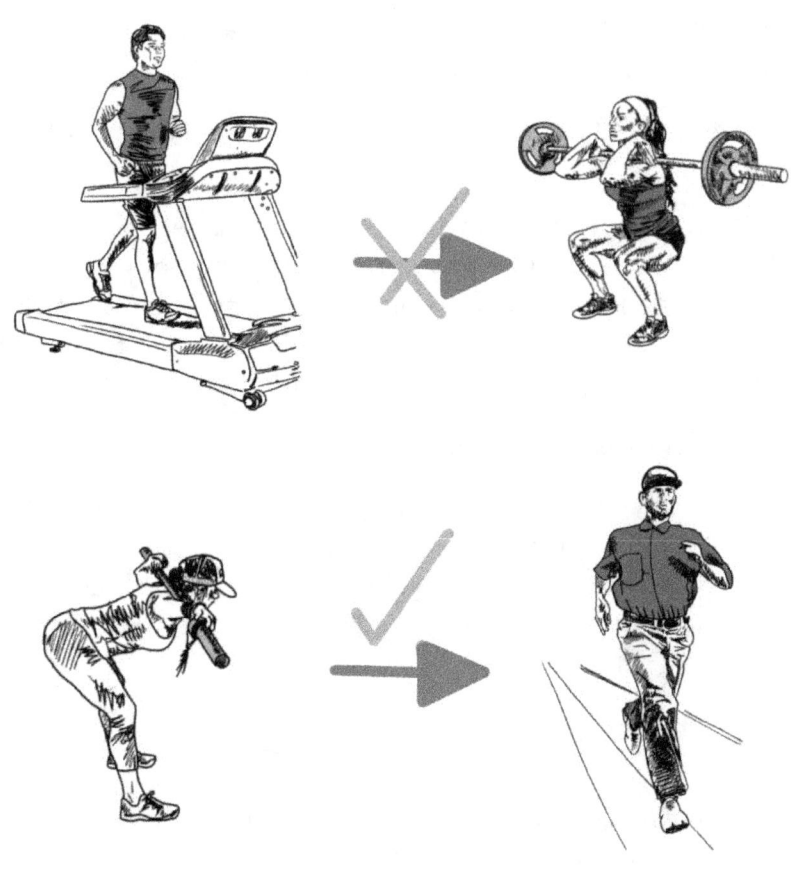

40. If you take a large grip on your Pull Ups, it will allow you to better target your lats muscles

"Is that true? Because I've always heard that if I took a larger grip, it could better recruit the lats muscle?"

So, a word of caution: Here I am not talking of a street workout goal where one of the goals is to go reach a maximum of repetitions on the pull up. In that case, one of the parameters will perhaps be to reduce the pulling range of motion of the athlete (and to analyse his competitors).

But the article here covers muscular recruitment. So, what about it?

It turns out that a study realised in 2014 analysed the topic[ix]. A team of Norwegian researchers tested 3 different grip widths on experienced weight training practitioners depending on their shoulder width as well as on an intensity relative to the maximal load they were able to move for each grip width.[49]

The results were irrevocable:

At a relatively identical intensity, no matter the grip width, muscle activation of the 4 observed muscles is similar during a high cable machine vertical pulldown. Moreover, the large grip does not allow to pull loads as heavy as close and medium grips.

---

[49] The research has been realised with the assistance of EMG. We must take into account that EMG (electromyography) are indicators but they do not predict hypertrophy. It nonetheless remains an interesting research paper.

Regarding close and medium grips, they recruit in an identical or just slightly superior manner the latissimus dorsi, the trapezoids, the infraspinatus and the brachii biceps. Moreover, the large grip does not allow to pull as heavy than close and medium grips (for the majority of athletes).

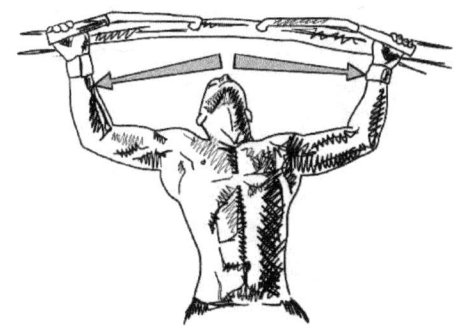

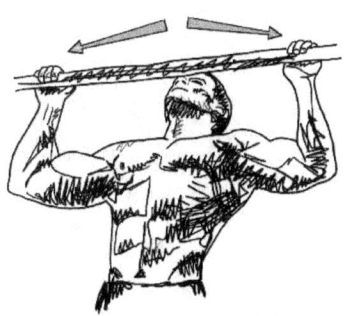

To be noted: with time, a large grip on pullups can increase joint constraints.

> Conclusion:
>
> A priori, a large grip does not possess real advantages compared with a close or medium grip. Favour the one which suits you best. Nonetheless, we can make a hypothesis regarding regional hypertrophy of the lats muscle fascicles. That could be interesting during a mechanical dropset or for another goal. It could be worth the cost adding some variety from time to time.

41. It burns so much! I am unable to finish my movement because of lactic acid!

It is a sentence frequently heard in gyms and in the world of running.

The burning sensation[lxi] is linked to muscular fatigue. It involves the accumulation of "chemical waste[50]" which occur during energy production. The more the effort is intense, the more the "waste" accumulates rapidly.

And lactic acid then? Is it really because of it that I am unable to finish my exercise?

This affirmation is impossible for the simple and good reason that the body has never produced lactic acid and that it probably never will.

So, what is it?

It is lactate. Lactate is a base rather than an acid.

Lactate is an energetic substrate[lxii]. It represents the final product of glycolysis[51] independently of the presence of oxygen. It can be used in the mitochondria[52].

---

[50] Metabolite accumulation: Metabolites are components produced by nutrients degradation. Their function is to provide the body with the type of energy it needs.

[51] Glycolysis is the degradation of glucose from a living being, under the action of enzymes.

[52] Mitochondria have the role of providing energy to cells, and that of allowing their survival and their functions.

<u>To be taken into account:</u>

It already occurred to me hearing that stretching allows eliminating lactic acid. Although, above, we have tried to explain that lactic acid is not viable in the human body, it should be noted that lactate (and so not lactic acid) is eliminated by the hepatic system and that it is not the cause of muscle soreness.[53]

Conclusion:

Lactic acid is not viable in the human body. Lactate is.

---

[53] Hepatic function is the array of actions performed by the liver. It essentially has 3 functions: the fabric and storage of energy, the fabric of bile, and detoxification (rendering harmless toxic products absorbed by the intestines).

42. Improve your muscle gains thanks to pre-exhaustion!

Pre-exhaustion consists of placing a single-joint exercise before a multi-joint exercise. The goal being to best recruit the "pre-exhausted" muscle.

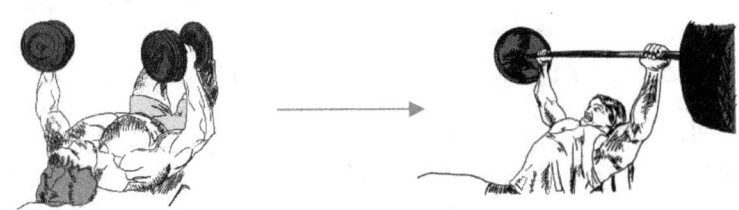

Apparently, this would be addressed to people who have difficulty feeling a muscle group on a polyarticular movement because adjunct muscles take the lead.

For example, triceps and shoulders "let go" before the pecs. The consequence being that we do not manage to finish our set on our bench press.

But what does science say?

At the time when these lines are written, there is little research[54] on pre-exhaustion but they do not go in the direction of the popular belief. In fact, in the realm of weight training, there does not seem to be advantages to using this method to develop a muscle or a muscle group.

---

[54] At the time being, two studies have been realised on novice individuals and one research has been realised on trained individuals.

A research paper would even seem to show that training volume, contrarily to what we could think, is diminished in a training using pre-exhaustion contrarily to a traditional training which does not make use of this type of method.

To be taken into account:

Adherence remains an important element in a weight training programme. If someone would like to add some pre-exhaustion as part of their programme, it would be wise to explain to that person that we can go in their way by taking into account their level according to what science tells us for the time being.

Another form of pre-exhaustion exists within the realm of physical preparation (outside of weight training)[lxiii]. That one has for goal to train the athlete to a state of fatigue close to the one encountered in a competition. It can be useful for disciplines which combine power and endurance.

Conclusion:

Pre-exhaustion in weight training does not go in the direction of the popular belief. At best, hypertrophy and muscle gains seem similar. At worse, that could prove itself counterproductive.

43. Base yourself on mind-muscle connection and on sensation to improve your muscle gains!

Very renown in the world of bodybuilding, is the famous mind-muscle connection based on science? Can we rely on it and use it to optimise our muscle gains?

Firstly, it is important to define what muscle-mind connection is.

Neuromuscular connection (mind-muscle)[55] is a sort of internal attention. Its goal is to direct all the athlete's attention and concentration on the muscle or the group of muscles at play in a well-defined strength training exercise. This internal focus opposes itself to external focus. External focus concentrates itself on 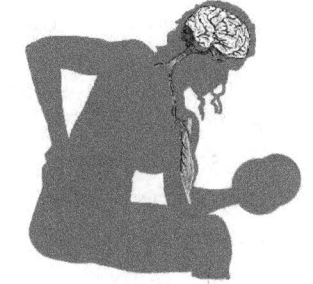 the movement and not on the muscle(s) involved.
It is important to already distinguish between different aspects before going further and making the links with the factor we would like to develop.[lxiv]

Concerning hypertrophy, it would appear that there is an improvement in muscle mass gains by using this internal focus technique.[lxv]

---

[55] Mind-muscle connection is a popularised term used to define the neuromuscular connexion (also named internal focus)

However, for the development of sports performances and of strength, an external focus seems to bring superior results.[lxvi]

On the other hand, mind-muscle connection has its limits. In fact, that one allows a muscular activation for intensities going from 20 to 60% of the RM, but at 80% of that one, there are no more differences.[lxvii] In addition, this internal focus shows effects on slow speeds of execution, but no difference on an elevated speed[lxviii]. Yet, concerning hypertrophy, we know that "tempo" does not bring significant differences for the development of muscle gains.[lxix]

Finally, mind-muscle connection allows for a better muscle activation at the start of a set, but the more we approach ourselves from muscle failure, the more the difference disappears.[lxx] Let's remind ourselves that the fact of getting close to muscle failure still remains an essential factor in hypertrophy.

It is also important to note that an internal focus can inhibit the economy of movement, and so, with time, deteriorate the technical gesture.

Conclusion:

Concerning hypertrophy, mind-muscle connection seems interesting in certain situations. Nonetheless, these situations in which we can find some value to it sometimes go against the foundations of hypertrophy like getting close to muscle failure and the execution tempos of the movement for example. With regards to strength development, concentrating ourselves on the movement (external focus) seems to optimise technique and lead to the obtention of better results. Internal focus, on its side, generally generates a co-contraction. It is as if we were loading "heavier" because the antagonist muscle produces additional tension.

44. A big back for a big bench press!

Some athletes of the powerlifting world and of the bench press world are not managing to reach an agreement on the topic.

Doe shaving a big back contribute to performance optimisation on the concentric phase for the Bench Press[56]?

It is important to first look back into the anatomical functions of the latissimus dorsi muscle, the trapezius muscle and the rhomboids muscle to understand their implication on the human body:

- The latissimus dorsi muscle allows: internal rotation and extension of the arms (in other words, it allows bringing the hand to the opposite buttock, whilst lowering the shoulder.), the back's curve and the lateral incline of the hips and inspiration.

- The rhomboids muscle allows: adduction, medial elevation and rotation of the scapula. By its effect of scapular rotation, it is a shoulder depressor.

- The trapezius muscle: The trapezius is divided into 3 parts. The upper fascicle allows shrugging our shoulders, extending our head backward and turning our head controlaterally[57] to the muscle, and inclining it homolaterally[58].

---

[56] We are here speaking of bench press with no equipment.

[57] Controlateral: Located on the opposite side.

[58] Homolateral: Which is located or which occurs on a same side of the body.

The medium fascicle, on his side, allows approaching the scapula to the spine and pulling the shoulder backwards. Finally, the inferior fascicle has for goal to lower the shoulders. The 3 fascicles allow stabilising the scapula.

- The erector spinae muscles: this is a group of muscles located at the bottom of the back which allows spinal extension.

After having analysed the main anatomical functions of the back muscles (there are others such as the infraspinatus, the supraspinatus, ...), what can we already say?

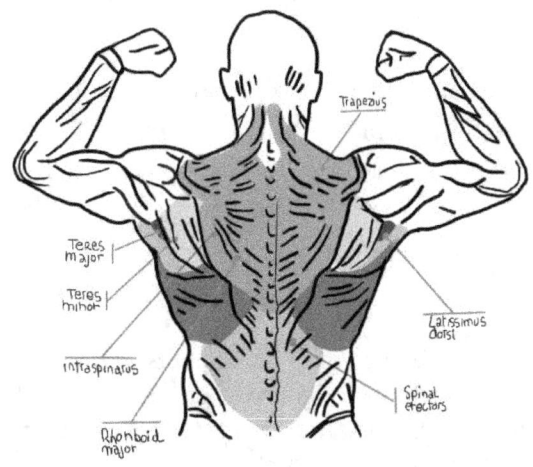

It would seem like there is a value in engaging the back on the bench press with the goal of stabilising the shoulders and of contributing to the movement's stability more generally.[lxxi] Nonetheless, it seems like the back muscles are not priority muscles for performance on the bench press.

And the science in all of that?

There are not many studies for the time being, but some have proven to be very interesting on the bench press and notably on the arch (lumbar curve) and on scapular retraction. The research[lxxii] notably had the goal of comparing powerlifting athletes[59] on a one-repetition maximum and the pace of execution between a bench press with a flat back and a slight scapular retraction during a bench press session and a bench press with a lumbar curve and a pronounced scapular retraction during another session. It turns out that by the end of the protocol, there were no notable differences on both of the factors analysed (the development of 1RM and the pace of execution).

Another study[lxxiii] aimed to check the differences in total load, bar path on the sagittal plane[60] and in terms of the bar's mean speed between arched and flat techniques on the bench press as it pertains to novice and experienced paralympic powerlifting athletes[61].

---

[59] The athletes made up for 11 participants with 4 to 5 years of experience and a mean body weight of 87kg. On average, their bench press represents 1,3 to 1,4 their body weight. It is a good performance but not exceptional for a powerlifting athlete.

[60] In anatomy, the saggital plane, or longitidunal plane, is an anatomical plane which divides the body in left or right parts. The plane can be at the centre of the body and divided into two halves or far from the median line and divided it into unequal parts.

[61] There were few age differences between the novice and experienced (34 to 36 years old) powerlifting athletes. In the research, we estimated that an experienced athlete was one with a practice of 9,8 months (on average) and a novice trainee was an athlete with an experience of 3,3 months on average.

Concerning the arched and flat techniques, there was no significant difference for all the results analysed during the eccentric and the concentric phases of the movement for the novice and for the experienced athletes. Nonetheless, the research considers that more in-depth studies are necessary to determine the best techniques for athletes.

<u>To be taken into account:</u>

The studies cited above have the tendency to oppose themselves to the popular belief that a good stability (with the help of a lumbar curve and an important scapular retraction) will necessarily allow improved performance on the bench press. We also have the right to question ourselves regarding the lack of technical optimisation in both techniques with a risk of bias[62]. It would be interesting to develop studies on powerlifting athletes with an international level and/ or on bench press athletes with an international level in order to know if that lumbar curve technique makes more sense depending on the level and on the weight indicated on the barbell, or not.

The popular belief supposes that the arch serves as a force transmitter between the upper and the lower limbs. It is also meant to reduce the movement's range of motion in order to have more maximum strength or, at least, more capabilities to produce more maximum strength. Still, to this day, it seems that there is no biomechanical calculation which supports these underpinnings.

---

[62] A bias is an approach or process which generates errors in a study's results.

> Conclusion:
>
> Having a "strong and muscular" back will not directly allow being stronger on your bench press. To be strong on a movement, you must practice it, and eventually, supplement it with other exercises by individualising the programme depending on the goal and the individual. Regarding stability on the bench press as it relates to the back muscles, the current research seems to prove the contrary, but other studies are necessary to support those ideas and add perspective to the popular belief.

PART 2: Fitness scams: Pointless devices and other hoaxes

"The bigger the scam and the more it goes about unobserved"
[Philippe Chavanis]

What revolts me the most in the fitness world are the lies. Mistakes are entirely excusable. I have made some and it is very likely that I will make some again. By the way, making some mistakes is a beneficial process for each individual's personal evolution when we get to understand that these were mistakes. Nonetheless, making some mistakes and repeating them several times without critically thinking about them denotes of profound stupidity.

There where I encounter real problems in the fitness industry relates to taking advantage of a sedentary and neophyte's population lack of judgement. Very often, this type of public engages in physical activity or sport because they have a trigger moment leading them to want to change things for their health. Selling a dream to this needy population by very well knowing that there is no guarantee of result, that, however, it scandalises me.

The worst, it is the profit made by certain influencers selling the product like a miracle recipe against cellulite, against back pain and so on. An influencer, like the name indicates it, has for role to influence. That can turn out to be treacherous for its community in certain situations.

Ladies and gentlemen,

For you, I blow down these products qualified as "miracle products" that we principally find in the fitness and wellness worlds which only have the goal of scamming people and taking away money without any guarantee behind them.

However, I will not cite any brand, any name and I will not showcase any product in this chapter in order to avoid any kind of appeal to the courts.

Are you ready? *Here we go!*

45. The posture shirt

Sold as being THE t-shirt to absolutely get hold of for back pain and validated by medicine.

It is a hoax.

Don't you find that strange that we are sold a product validated by medicine but unfindable in a pharmacy?'

"Well, well, well…"

I went a bit further in my research to know what that was all about. And here is what I've found via a few scientific studies[lxxiv] :

- There is absolutely no difference between a classic t-shirt and a "posture shirt"

- The bad posture doesn't "really" exist. The human being is not made to constantly remain in a static position, he is made to move.

- There is no difference concerning the famous shoulders forward between a postural shirt and a classic t-shirt

In addition, the "posture shirt" is expensive (sometimes above 100€!). If you are still thinking of investing in this type of t-shirt, you should rather donate your money to an organisation which fights for peace in the world or to help needy people. At least, you'd engage in a good action and will not throw your money out the window.

Conclusion:

There is no advantage in buying a posture shirt. It is a loss of money. The treatment first starts with you and your profound capacity to want to change and to evolve. That could potentially be worse because we could suppose that the posture shirt leads our muscles to relax as we take it off as there would be less support.

46. Push Ups board

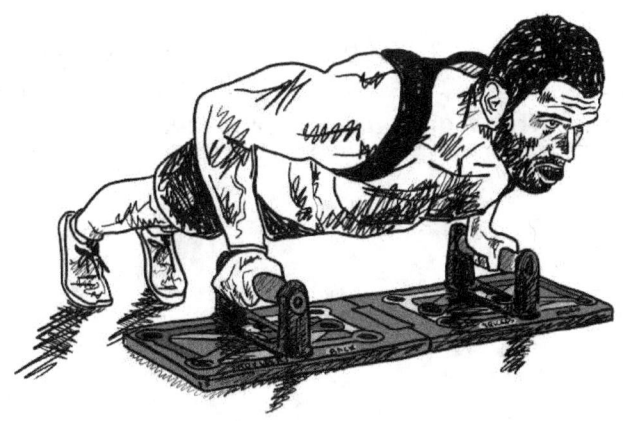

Although some boards have an integrated system which allows counting repetitions, how are they validated? There is nothing which indicates that your push up is well executed.

In addition, the board indicates you where to position your wrists thanks to colours codes (most of the time). Although that resembles more a Tetris than anything else, it does not take into account the physiology of the individual. The Push Ups board dimensions completely ignores whether you measure 1m60 or 2m10. It also ignores your eventual pathologies.

Last negative point: the price. It remains expensive for what it's worth (between 14€ and 60€ la most of the time).

In short, if you want to invest in some equipment to improve your push ups, favour simple Push Ups handles. They are not cumbersome; you can take them with you everywhere and they are less expensive (you have the possibility to find some between 9€ and 15€. (Sometimes even less expensive than those prices)!

> Conclusion:
>
> If you need to invest in material to improve the difficulty of your push ups, come back to the basics and favour Push Ups handles. No need to invest in gadgets with extravagant prices.

47. The legging & the anti-cellulite suction cup

Once again, influencers and fitness businesses take advantage of individuals concerned by their physical appearance, and it is truly scandalous.

As explained in the article 28 of the first chapter "Myths and popular beliefs", there is no treatment to make cellulite definitely disappear. Having cellulite is natural.

No matter the treatment or the product that you will use, this will not change anything on the long term. Scientific research has proven it by the way.

Conclusion:

Accept yourself as you are, there is no miracle products to efficiently treat cellulite on the long term and make it disappear.

---

48. The sweat belt

Be it in movies or in the gym, we have already encountered this famous cliché of the guy (it can also be a woman but it is seldom) who is on his treadmill with his coat and who is sweating so bad that he looks like the Niagara Falls. As you ask him why he imposes that upon himself, there are strong chances that the answer will be "to lose weight".

So, the sweat belt/ jumpsuit. Is if effective to lose fat?

Of course, I leaned on the question, by questioning different coaches and athletes of the Belgian capital to add additional knowledge to my expertise.

The question was simple: Are you for or against the sweat belt to lose fat?

Here are some of the different extracts:

The viewpoint of a CrossFit athlete previously a CrossFit coach:

"The question is not for or against the sudation belt but rather for or against weight loss thanks to this belt. I am totally against because unfortunately it doesn't lead to weight loss but only water loss. In fact, we lose water, so we have the impression of accelerating our weight loss but the water loss is momentary. When we are thirsty, we drink in order to fill in a deficit. It is what happens after a physical effort to counter the phenomenon of dehydration. That sudation is however very useful to eliminate the toxins depending on the manufacturer but this remains to be verified."

Viewpoint of a physical trainer and bodybuilding athlete:

"Against. Because firstly, a sweat or jumpsuit belt only leads to water loss and not fat loss like the majority imagine, which will directly be put back on once we start drinking again. In addition, more water loss means a decrease in performance, so a lower quality training.

Secondly, the jumpsuit impedes the body from properly making use of its thermoregulation system via sweat since the suit impedes the contact between the air and the skin. So, increase in body temperature. And so, once again, there will be a reduction in performance..."

Same story with the viewpoint of a third coach specialised in cross training:

"As far as I'm concerned, the sweat belt is big nonsense! You basically lose water, not body fat, and if you do too much you end up dehydrated so it is not very suggested. If the sweat belt really worked, putting it without doing any effort would be enough, but unfortunately it is not sweat which leads to weight loss but physical activity. So, for me it is just a scam for desperate souls which absolutely want to lose weight."

Viewpoint from instructor Wing Chun:

"Personally, I am neither for nor against. It doesn't help losing weight. It helps in losing water via the sweat induced which we recover quite rapidly once we hydrate. However, it could have a motivating effect for the individual wearing it. If it pushes the individual to surpass himself, why not."

Same story from a physical trainer specialised in the domains of powerlifting and weightlifting, also having a similar viewpoint on the question:

"We know that sweating doesn't increase caloric expenditure. Yet, it is admitted that whatever the training and nutrition methods used, weight loss always results from the fact that we have a negative calorie balance. Or more precisely, that the individual expends more energy than he is consuming. In addition, we will remember that water is at the core of multiple biochemical reactions in the body, and accelerating dehydration via a belt whilst most people aren't drinking enough is quite a bad idea.

We could think that the sweat belt and jumpsuit can be useful for an athlete who needs to attain his category's weight for a competition. But no, the sauna and the waterload remain much more appreciable methods."

My personal viewpoint converges with all the preceding viewpoints. There is no real benefit in using this type of method. After having discussed with MMA fighters, a point has retained my attention. The sudation belt could serve a purpose to prepare to a combat in a country where temperatures are elevated to get used to sensations and not be surprised by the D-day. But that represents a negligible part of the population.

Conclusion:

The sweat belt has no utility for weight loss. It is a useless marketing tool for most of the population.

49. The weight loss Hula Hoop

Honestly there... I don't have the words! To tell you everything, I didn't know we were able to get that far on the commercial side.

For the Hula Hoop, I discovered that by watching youtube where an influencer uses it and boasts about its merits without real convictions.

Apparently, the Hula Hoop allows for an "easy rotation" thanks to a centrifugal ball to lose weight effortlessly.

If you lose weight, it is not thanks to a magical device, but rather by training methods and by physical activity as well as an appropriate diet.

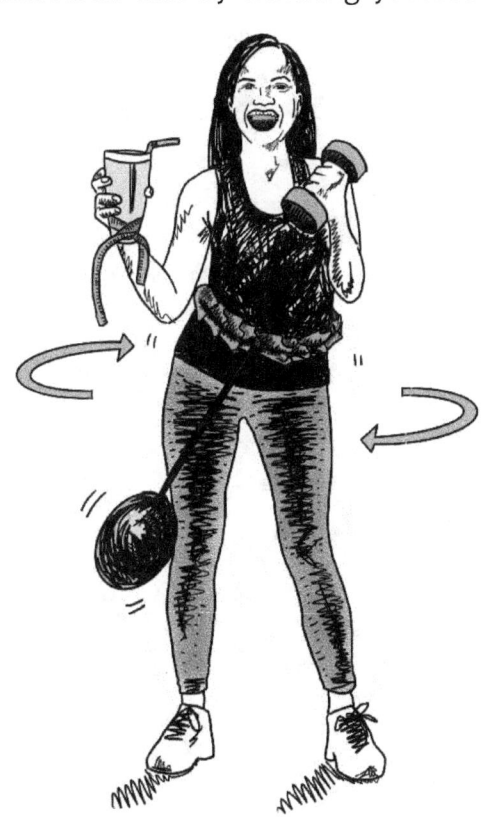

> Conclusion:
>
> It is not the device which will make you lose weight, but physical activity will.

50. The Facial Toner

I didn't even know that existed! I discovered this thing via an influencer.

The "Facial Toner" is a piece of rubber that you put in the mouth and with which you divert yourself by chewing it. Quite simply.

No really, I swear, it is not a joke.

The goal? Making the traits of the jaw prominent. It would apparently make you sexy.

The price? Between 2€ and 30€, sometimes even more!

In brief, take a chewing gum or eat a steak, it will be just the same.

Conclusion:

You already use your jaw naturally whilst eating. In addition, when you eat, you do not look like a dog which bites in a bone, contrarily to using this piece of rubber.

51. The double chin mask

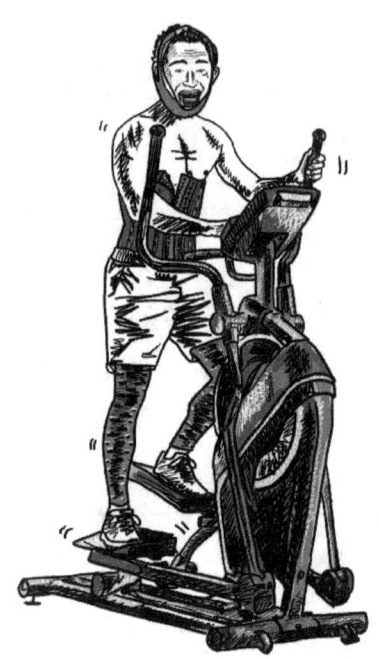

What annoys me is the mention "clinically proven" that certain products indicate in their descriptions. When we start doing research related to the proof that this works, it is very difficult to find results.

Nonetheless, I found an article of which the author is David Picovski, qualified by the Order of Doctors in plastic, repair and aesthetic Surgery ("l'Ordre des Médecins en Chirurgie plastique, réparatrice et esthétique" in French).

By searching for the causes of the double chin in the article, here is what comes out:

It can be due to aging, to skin sagging and to fat mass accumulation.

Apart for exceptions requiring a more in-depth treatment, the principal cause of the double chin is weight-related.

What annoys me is the term "slimming mask" used on internet. "Slimming" means which "leads to weight loss".

As specified previously (see article 4) and, by the way, proved scientifically[lxxv], fat loss is not targetable. Consequently, how is it possible to lose fat in a localised way, and that, in a clinically proved manner?

Conclusion:
Losing the double chin in a localised manner is impossible.

52. The vibration plate

The use of the vibration plate was trendy in fitness gyms some time ago, and it has now almost disappeared, Internet or teleshopping set aside when they propose it.

So... Does it really work?

Alors... Est-ce que ça marche vraiment ?

Here is what comes out from many comparative studies[lxxvi] between a training with a vibration plate and a classical training:

Regarding strength and power:

No significant improvements between a classic training and a training on a vibration plate.

Regarding speed:

No notable improvement on speed as compared to a classical training.

Regarding bone mineral density:

Training with a vibration plate allows increasing bone mineral density, but it only represents one of the recommended physical activities amongst others for the treatment of osteoporosis. Training with a vibration plate can complement postmenopausal treatment methods already known and bring tangible results in therapy.

The price varies between 80 and 500 € (sometimes more).

To be taken into consideration:

It is now well established that being exposed to vibrations can lead to harmful effects. According to OSHA (Occupational & Safety Hazard Association), a long-term exposition to vibrations can also provoke nausea, visual disturbances, hyperventilation and disorders such as the Raynaud's Syndrome, the Hand-arm vibration Syndrome and the Carpal Tunnel Syndrome.[lxxvii]

Nonetheless, we are all different. Consequently, we must also understand that the frequency, the intensity and the duration of the vibrations will be harmful for one individual and perhaps not for another.

In short, the vibration plate can be interesting to complement a treatment (e.g. osteoporosis) depending on certain patients' preferences, but it does not bring a radical change to the majority of performance-related factors in comparison to a classical weight training session in a gym. In addition, the price can turn out to be a notable budget for certain people.

Conclusion:

No significant differences between a classic training and a training with a vibration plate. In addition, vibration plates can turn out to be harmful in certain instances.

53. The stepper

The stepper has been put forward on television channels where it was presented like a revolutionary equipment.

Don't you see?

It is a little platform a little bigger than a shoe box (okay, let's say 2 shoe boxes!) on which we placed our feet on top and for which the functioning was the same as using pedals.

Well, concerning the calorie countdown that the stepper can indicate… We already know that there are high chances that the energy expenditure indicated on a fitness machine will be flawed[63].

We won't bite in the hand that feeds you too fast, but honestly, before buying a stepper… There still is the possibility to use something else and that without spending a single euro, no?

There have been a few studies[lxxviii] on the stepper in order to know if there was a major difference between using the stairs or a stepper in terms of muscle activation.

The result? No major difference.

The stepper and climbing stairs both allow reinforcing the knee extensor.[lxxix]

And the price? It varies between 40€ and 100 €.

---

[63]   See article 37 – Chapter 1

In short, next time, apart from specific pathologies, take the stairs.

And if you really want a stepper, favour a simple "step". It is a more versatile tool which doesn't require any batteries to function.

To be taken into consideration:

The stepper has shown beneficial impacts on the hip extensors in a specific context for individuals affected by a CVA (Cerebrovascular Accident) and under specific conditions in terms of support (mirroirs and preventive support). Nonetheless, that concerns a targeted public which goes beyond the scope cited.[lxxx]

> Conclusion:
>
> Apart from eventual pathologies, favour the stairs or a classic step. It is less expensive, and in the case of the classic step, it is more versatile for the exercises (Lunges, Push Ups with hands, elevated, etc.).

54. The meal replacement shake

As previously mentioned, I will not cite any brands.

Certain brands released a shake which would serve as a meal substitute. This means that it can replace a meal.

A shake which would apparently bring multiple vitamins and minerals necessary for the body's good functioning.

The little "+" of this drink? In addition to replacing a meal, it would allow us to save time in our day and reduce stress.

I would now like to come back to one of the jaw's main roles: chewing food.

Even though the shake can contain certain "pieces" (which must not render things very pleasant), I strongly doubt that chewing's role is well used.

And what is the purpose of chewing?

According to certain articles and exchanges[lxxxi] with individuals specialised in nutrition, here is what chewing contributes to:

- It helps reducing digestive issues such as gastric refluxes, bloating, flatulence and stomach aches

- Reducing pressure on the sphincter of the oesophagus

- A good mastication also increases saliva production ensuring a better oral hygiene since saliva can neutralise certain bacteria

- Importance in weight management in that it allows better identifying hunger and fullness cues.

By the way, some studies have confirmed that chewing could contribute to diminishing the risk of developing obesity[lxxxii].

Well, now… Let's get back to the main advantages of the shake as stated by the companies' founder of this product of which we cannot pronounce the name:

- Replacing a meal by lack of time and being less stressed to keep control over our day

- Losing weight (slimming diet)

Have you not already heard or read a healthcare professional telling you that it is important to take the time to eat?

I completely agree upon the fact that we are today in a world in which everything is going very fast and that finding some time for little life pleasures is not always simple, and that it requires an adjustment of priorities.

Nonetheless, here are the problems we can run into when we eat too fast in order to have more time on your planning of the day:

- Digestive issues

- Satiety-related issues[64] and weight gain

These are the two major problems which are put forward the most according to studies and certain specialists say that it could even lead to sleep and mood disorders!

---

64   Satiety: State of someone which is completely satiated

In short, what is meant to allow you to enter a virtuous circle puts you more at risk of entering a vicious cycle. A shake should not replace a meal; however, it could turn out to be an interesting supplement in certain situations. Bref, ce qui est censé vous faire rentrer dans un cercle vertueux risque plutôt de vous faire rentrer dans un cercle vicieux. In addition to that, the price of certain supplements can prove to be very expensive.

To be taken into account:

In certain situations, a "processed and ultra-processed" diet can be interesting. For example, a patient suffering with malnutrition can use this solution. Everything is not to be rejected neither.

Conclusion:

A shake should be seen as a nutritional supplement and not as a meal substitute. First learn to eat well before turning to processed foods.

PART 3 : "The VERSUS"

"Of course, subtility is needed; but ensure that it is obvious."
[Billy Wilder]

Many individuals I supervise as part of my coachings asked numerous times the question:

"Why this variation of an exercise and not another?"

This question is totally legitimate as the individual that we supervise should know where she is heading in terms of goals. We must know how to answer to the needs but also to the questions of the athlete/ client.

In that part, I put forward alternatives to different exercises and provide you with an explanation regarding their recruitment, hoping that this will be helpful to you and that it will guide you in your trainings.

55. Axle Bar Deadlift VS Olympic Bar Deadlift

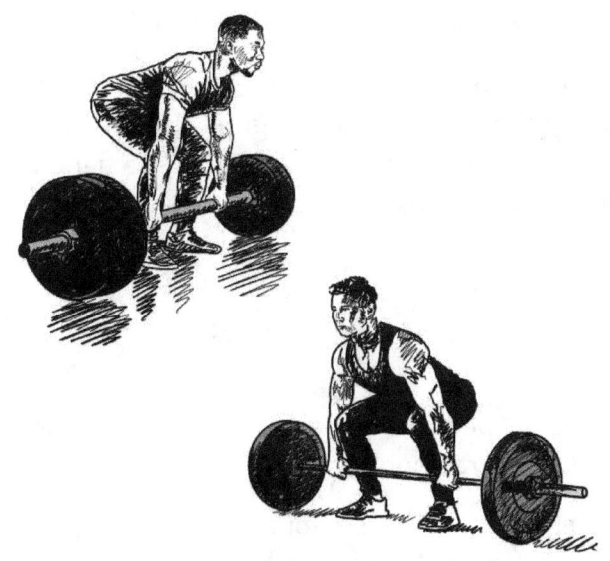

Before debating on the topic, it is important to understand what we are talking about (logical).

Here, we do not add a variation to the exercise itself, but to the equipment used.

The axle bar, also known under the name of fat bar, is very renown in the Strongman world. Its particularity, contrarily to an Olympic barbell ("classical" barbell that we find in weight training gyms) is its diameter. In fact, this one will be larger than that of a "classical" barbell, which will put your grip to the test.

But in the case of the Deadlift, what is the benefit of working with an axle Bar?

There is not only one benefit, but there are many benefits.

According to Charles Poliquin, pioneer in physical preparation and in strength development, working with thicker barbells allows a greater activation of motor units. More particularly, fibres of fast contraction.

But that is not all. A scientific study struck my attention concerning the work with "fat grip" (thickness of grip). This research involved analysing the effects of a tighter grip on the performances of division I golfers[lxxxiii] on a period of 8 weeks.

The results were surprising:

- Significant improvement of grip strength with a larger grip

- Overall better transference on the sporting discipline contrarily to a traditional training.

Nonetheless, that tool asks for a certain training experience as an athlete before being able to use it. In addition, we are speaking of one study only.

Although all gyms (unfortunately) do not dispose of an axle bar, it is possible to find some "fat grips" at a reasonable price. These are grips which are to be inserted on a barbell or on some dumbells, and which will allow having a larger grip for your trainings.

Concerning fat grips[lxxxiv], a study used this tool on trained men to examine its effects on muscle activation and on strength. The athletes had the goal of realising a one-repetition maximum with an Olympic bar on the deadlift, the bent over row, the upright row, the concentration curl (biceps curl with the elbow supported by the leg) and performing a set of pull ups to failure. The athletes had to realise this protocol with the fat grips and without the fat grips.

Everything was measured with EMG[65] data. What we have been able to observe is that the 1RM strength[66] was strongly diminished with the fat grips and so was the number of repetitions maximum on the pull ups. In contrast, electromyographic muscle activation was significantly increased in the forearm and shoulder muscles, but significantly diminished in the arm muscles with the use if the fat grip during the deadlift, the rowing and the pull ups. However, there was no difference for the upright row and for the concentration curl exercises. The differences in maximum strength, on pull ups performances and on EMG activity via the use of fat grips can be due to different muscle length positions. Although the fat grip training could increase neuromuscular activation, the study tends to indicate us that a reduction in muscular strength can lead to the prescription of low training loads which might not be ideal to develop muscular strength.

To be taken into account:

- Grip strength is an indicator of sarcopenia[67] prevention.

- Numerous studies have also wanted to analyse the effects of isometric work on cardio-vascular health.

---

[65] As a reminder, EMG (electromyographic activity) data are indicators, but, that said, they do not predict hypertrophy

[66] RM = A one-repetition maximum

[67] Sarcopenia: progressive and elevated loss of mass, of strength and of muscular functions with the aging process

Based on individual data, the principal results of this meta-analysis showed that isometric training allows diminishing arterial systolic[68], diastolic[69], and mean pressures in a significant manner. Strictly speaking, this does not involve work done with the axle bar or with fat grips, but fat grips can be interesting tools since they can generally be performed anywhere, at any time, in a sitting position, and they are easily accessible for every public, notably for people who have mobility issues (or a certain medical history/ pathologies) who could not immediately start by a cardiovascular training programme (walking, running, biking, swimming, etc.) or by a strength training programme. A few dozens of minutes per week of isometric work on maximum 1 or 2 exercises done at relatively low intensity (20-30% of maximum voluntary contraction) are sufficient to bring clinical benefits regarding the health status of individuals suffering from hypertension[lxxxv].

- A research[lxxxvi] realised a strength grip test of the hand. This one proved to be a reliable indicator of the body's general strength among the general population. This study aimed to determine whether the hand's grip test was a valid predictor of strength among a population of competitive powerlifters[70].

---

[68] Systolic blood pressure is the value of the pressure in the artery when the heart contracts itself.

[69] Diastolic pressure corresponds to the value of the pressure in the artery when the heart is at rest in-between two contractions.

[70] The subjects were competitive powerlifters registered to a competition on the State level. Measures related to size, to weight, to body composition and to grip strength were taken before the start of the competition.

The competitors participated either equipped, either non-equipped on the squat, the bench press and the deadlift. The results of the research suggest that grip strength is a good indicator of body total strength for non-equipped competitive powerlifters.

> Conclusion:
>
> Working with some "fat grips" seems beneficial in certain situations. Tools like the fat grip or the axle bar can be useful in the case of mitigating risks related to cardio-vascular diseases. Training grip strength is not to be neglected but it should not alter the main goal.

56. Front Squat VS Back Squat (high bar)

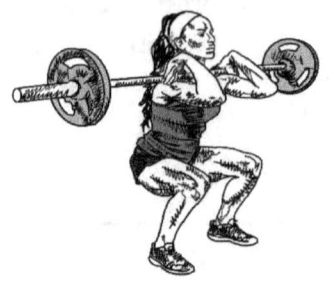

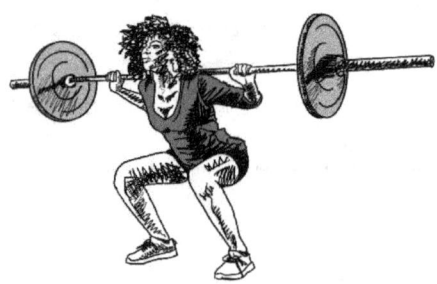

Without the shadow of a doubt, the "duel" which comes around the most. Very certainly the most well-known of all individuals involved in weight training.

The main difference? The repartition of the load. On the Back Squat, the bar is positioned "behind" you. On the Front Squat, on the other hand, it is positioned in front of you.

Concretely, what does it change?

According to EMG (electromyography) research and analyses, here is what comes out:

- The Front Squat allows a better activation of the quadriceps as a whole contrarily to the Back Squat.[lxxxvii] This can be explained by the different incline of the chest in the two movements.

- The Back Squat and the Front Squat have a similar activation of the hamstrings. Very slightly superior for the Back Squat but not in a significant manner (regardless of the depth of the work).[lxxxviii]

- The Back Squat generally requires less mobility than the Front Squat on the scapular belt.

- The Le Front Squat allows for a reduction of lumbar stress as compared to the Back Squat.

- The Front Squat allows a weaker knee compression than the Back Squat.[lxxxix]

If we look at all the benefits of the Front Squat regarding the recruitment of quadriceps muscles, we could think that it is an exercise which would remind us of the goose that lays golden eggs. And yet…

There is a difference between studies and field. One does not go without the other of course, but certain things must be taken into consideration:

- If you have some pain on the collarbone on the Front Squat and that you do not correctly place the bar on yourself, this can negatively impact the final result.

- Even on some Front Squat, if you incline your chest forward too much, the results will be altered in terms of quadriceps recruitment and it would then be better to perform some Zercher Squat or some Back Squat with elevated heels[71].

---

[71] Zercher Squat & Back Squat with elevated heels: here are only two examples among a multitude of potential solutions.

- If you lack shoulder mobility and have tensions towards your lower back, the Suitcase Squat/Farmer Squat with elevated heels can be an interesting alternative for you as well.

> Conclusion:
>
> The Front squat best recruits the quadriceps and brings less knee compression than the Back Squat. Nonetheless, if the exercise is not well executed, these results can be altered.

57. Hip Thrust VS Conventional Deadlift

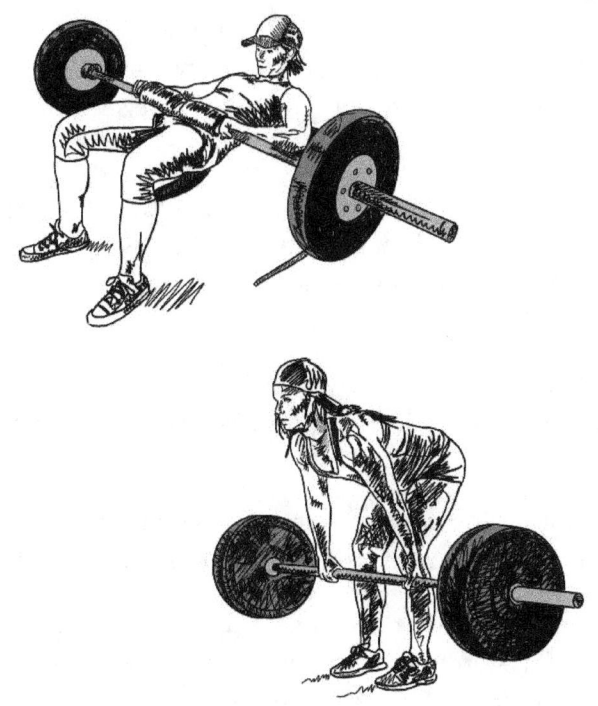

We know that the Hip Thrust and the Conventional Deadlift[72] (with an Olympic barbell) mostly target the posterior chain. Nonetheless, a few differences are to be taken into account:

-   The Hip Thrust is a good isolation exercise which allows maximising the contraction of the gluteus maximus muscles towards the end of the concentric phase The glutes recruitment is slightly superior than on the Deadlift.[x]

---

[72] Conventional Deadlift: traditional Deadlift

The Hip Thrust's lever arm is less important than that of the Deadlift for the lower back and the hips.

- The Deadlift allows a better hamstrings recruitment than the Hip Thrust, and that, in a significant manner, with a lighter load than the Hip Thrust exercise (difference of approximatively 20%)

- The difference in terms of recruitment of the biceps femoris (hamstring muscle) between the Olympic Deadlift and the Hip Thrust is principally due to the start of the concentric phase

- The Hip Thrust allows loading relatively heavy without requiring a technical learning process as important as for the Deadlift

- The Hip Thrust allows significantly improving performances with a horizontal direction (e.g. sprint)[xci]

- No significant difference between the Hip Thrust and the Deadlift regarding the recruitment of the spinal erectors on the different phases of the movement

---

Conclusion:

The Hip Thrust totally has its place in physical preparation and it has shown serious benefits for horizontal direction performances. It increases the recruitment of glutes to work the posterior chain contrarily to its Deadlift counterpart. Nonetheless, the Deadlift allows a better recruitment of the biceps femoris.

58. Pull Ups (pronated) VS Chin Ups (supinated)

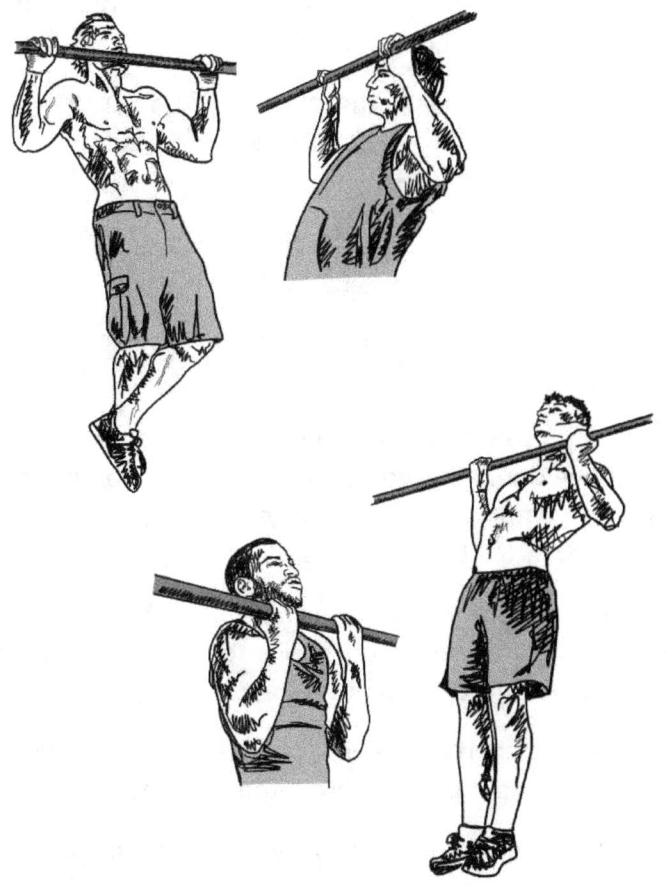

"Coach why do we use that kind of grip?"

It is a question which comes back frequently and it is normal to ask it!

I haven't put forward the neutral grip Pull Up (also called the "Perfect Pull Ups") but I will mention that one in this article.

Between Chin Ups and Pull Ups[xcii], there is a difference in terms of muscle recruitment concerning the biceps brachi, the lower trapezius and the pectoralis major.

- There is no major difference concerning the recruitment of the latissimus dorsi or that of the spinal erectors between the two versions of the Pull Up

- The pectoralis major and the biceps brachi (arm) are more engaged during the supinated Pull Ups

- The lower trapezius is more engaged during the pronated Pull Ups

What is important to understand, and that, by the way, I have myself done during my coachings, is that it is possible to adapt the grip depending on an injury and to keep an "equivalent" recruitment of the back muscles.

Concerning neutral grip Pull Ups for which I have not done the comparison compared to the supinated and the pronated Pull Ups, it should be known that they allow:

- A better recruitment of the latissimus dorsi[xciii] (as compared to supinated and pronated Pull Ups)

- A similar recruitment of the pectoralis major compared to supinated Pull Ups.

– A superior recruitment of the rear delt as compared to the supinated grip.

I see you coming… So, I anticipate!

"Oh well if the supinated grip is easier for me coach, why don't you put it in my programme since the recruitment of the back muscles is similar?"

It is logical, I don't blame you. Here is my answer:

Although getting too close of the sport's gesture in a specific way is not my approach of physical preparation and of coaching (I think that diversifying the sport's gesture will have a greater advantage for the athlete, but it all depends on the context and the period). We must not find ourselves on the opposite spectrum either. We must keep in mind that a certain similarity of daily situations that we can find in daily life or in a sporting discipline has its importance.

What's better than illustrating it with a few examples?

Have you already seen a climbing athlete climb with a supinated grip?

Have you already seen a street lifting athlete perform the heaviest Muscle Up possible with a supinated grip during a competition?

Have you already seen a CrossFit athlete perform some Kipping Pull Ups with a supinated grip?

It is very rare to be able to overcome an obstacle with a supinated grip.

Conclusion:

Regardless of the grip used, the recruitment of the back muscles is similar between the supinated and the pronated grips on the Pull Ups. The supinated grip will allow a better recruitment on the biceps brachii whereas the pronated grip will allow a better recruitment of the lower trapezius.

59. Reverse Hyperextension VS Back Extension

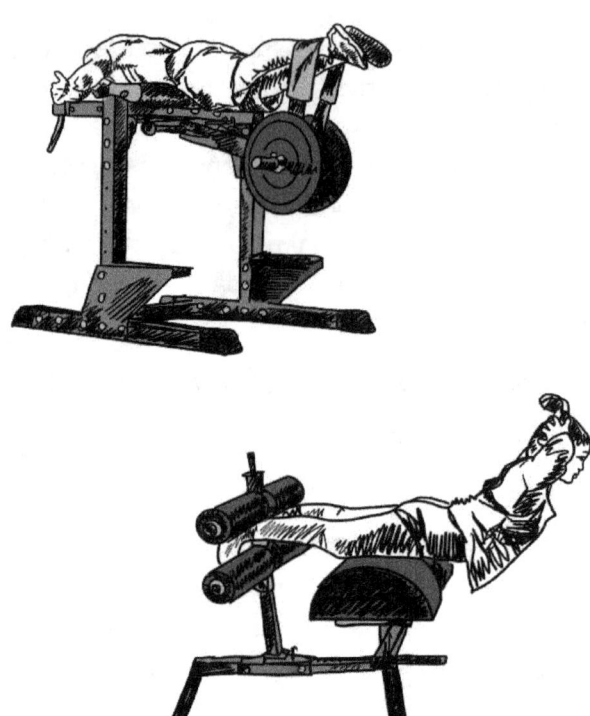

Here we have two similar exercises which nonetheless differ in many respects, and that's what we will take a closer look at.

The Back Extension is more popularised in CrossFit and in traditional strength training gyms than the Reverse Hyperextension.

The Reverse Hyperextension was popularised by Louie Simmons from Westside Barbell. According to him, the Reverse Hyperextension would allow a decompression of the lower part of the spine.

But in what do they differ? A study[xciv] compared both fitness tools whilst keeping the same work load for the Back Extension and for the Reverse Hyperextension.

- The Back Extension allows a better activation of the glute max and of the biceps femoris (hamstrings) than the Reverse Hyperextension.

- The Reverse Hyperextension allows a longer time with a lower back extension thanks to a larger level arm. However, this does not bring more muscle activation as compared to the Back Extension.

- The Back Extension possesses a less important range of motion between the thigh and the trunk as compared to the Reverse Hyperextension.

- The Reverse Hyperextension brings a weaker lumbar flexion than the Back Extension

- The Reverse Hyperextension allows stimulating the muscles in the same manner whilst offering a larger range of motion towards the hips and by reducing that one towards the lumbar zone

To be taken into account:

Researchers have equalised the loads between both exercises. Yet, as a result of the momentum during the Reverse Hyperextension, it will probably be more interesting to add load on that exercise. Louie Simmons generally suggests loading to a value equivalent to 50% of the load used during your sets of squat[xcv].

> Conclusion:
>
> The Reverse Hyperextension allows diminishing the lumbar flexion whilst increasing the movement's range of motion at the hip. It therefore allows stimulating the muscles in the same manner (in comparison to the Back Extension) and offers a greater range of motion at the hips whilst reducing the range of motion towards the lumbar zone.

60. Good Morning VS Deadlift

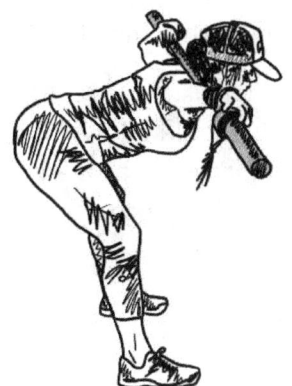

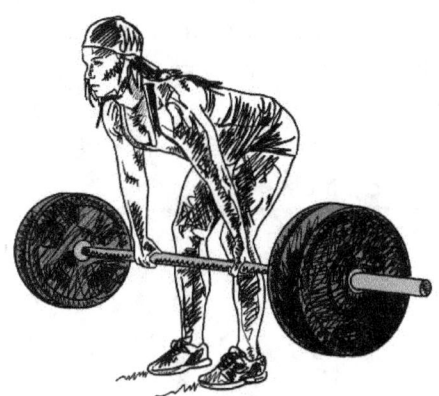

The movements are similar but the distribution of the load is different. The Good Morning is an exercise sometimes left behind in weight training gyms. Still, is it useless compared to the Deadlift? That is what we will see:

-       The Deadlift and the Good Morning both allow recruiting the hamstrings, the glutes, the lower back and the adductors.

-       The Deadlift allows having a higher load than the Good Morning due to the distribution of the load in relation to the body.

- To considerably reduce the risk of injury linked to a rupture of the anterior cruciate ligament (ACL), the researchers suggest practising the Good Morning rather than the Deadlift[xcvi]

- The Good Morning uses a smaller range of motion towards the hip and the knee. This would allow for a better recruitment of the hamstrings compared to a Deadlift in the case where the load would be identical on both exercises.[xcvii]

Conclusion:

In the context of reducing the risk of injury linked to a rupture of the ACL, the Good Morning is more interesting than the Deadlift. For powerlifting, CrossFit and weight lifting athletes mainly, the Good Morning can be interesting in addition to their main exercises, but the Deadlift remains essential to perform in those disciplines.

61. Shoulder Press (Barbell) VS Shoulder Press (Dumbbells)

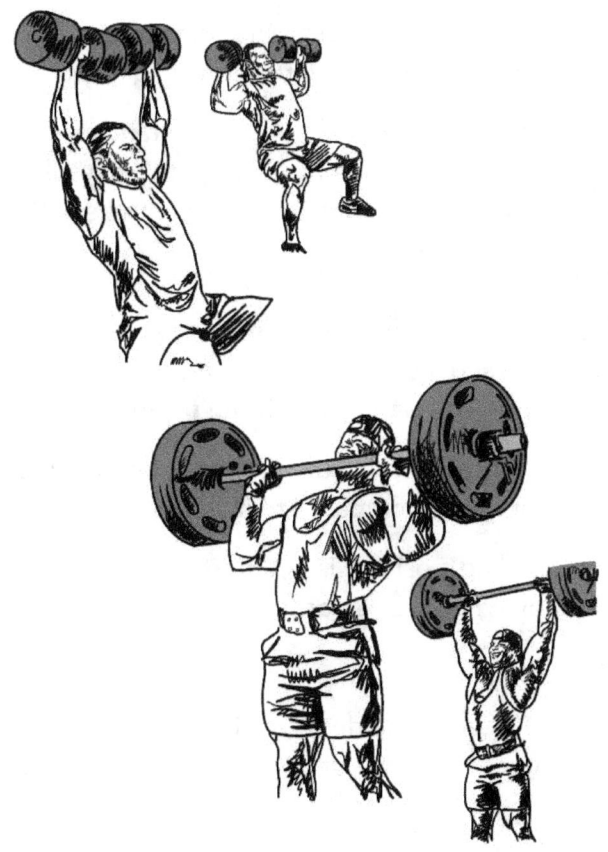

The Shoulder Press is an exercise which aims to develop the shoulder muscles.

But what is the most effective version in terms of muscle activation?

To know it, a scientific research[xcviii] compared the dumbbells and barbell Shoulder Press exercise, also doing so by varying the starting positions (standing and sitting).

Here is what comes out of it:

For the anterior delt:

- Sitting position: The dumbbells Shoulder Press has a superior activation of 11% in comparison to the Barbell Shoulder Press

- The standing dumbbells Shoulder Press has an 8% superior activation compared with the sitting position

- The dumbbells Shoulder Press in standing position is significantly superior (15%) compared to the barbell Shoulder Press in standing position as it pertains to muscle activation

For the side delt:

- The barbell Shoulder Press has a 7% superior neuromuscular activation when this one is performed in a standing position compared to a sitting position.

- When it is performed standing, the dumbbells Shoulder Pres sis 7% superior as compared to its barbell counterpart.

- The standing position is 15% better compared with the sitting position when we perform the exercise with dumbbells.

For the rear delt:

- The dumbbells Shoulder Press in standing position is 24% superior compared with the sitting position with dumbbells.

To be taken into account:

Contrarily to the dumbbells, the barbell allows carrying heavier loads on the long term, but this requires a certain level.

What is important to take into account in this research is neuromuscular activation. It seems that we benefit of a greater activation of a posture with less stability. Yet, we know that instability is quite a disadvantage for hypertrophy.

Conclusion:

According to this research, the dumbbells Shoulder Press in standing position allows the best neuromuscular activation for the whole shoulder. However, this does not seem to be the most suitable solution for the development of strength and of hypertrophy. En revanche, cela ne semble pas être la solution la plus adaptée pour le développement de la force et de l'hypertrophie. In that perspective, it would be wiser to favour a stable surface and to apply the basics of progressive overload.

62. Running on a treadmill VS Running outside

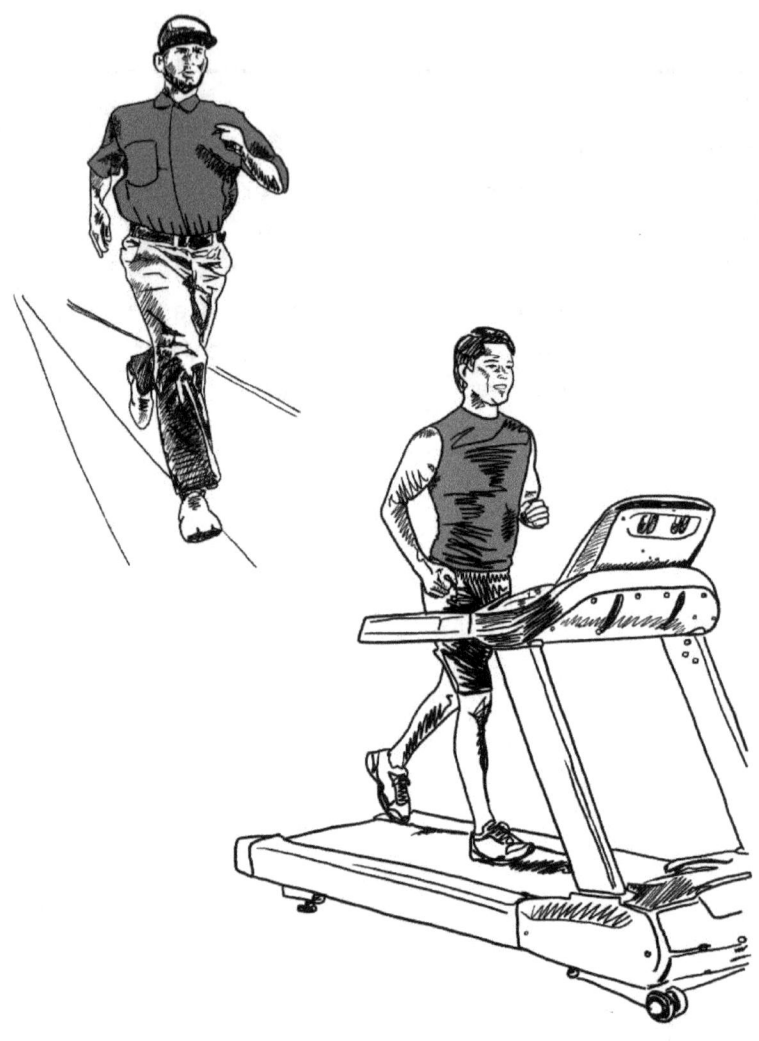

We will not beat around the bush and so we will directly give you the best alternative! Go run outside!

Why?

- It is free (well yes, it is an advantage!)

- Running outside expends more calories than running on a treadmill (about 10% more)

Why is that?

In an outside setting, we are confronted to certain parameters that we do not find at the gym:

- The weather (e.g. wind)

- The slopes

- The surfaces (rocky, muddy, etc)

This will therefore require more effort than on a treadmill, and so (potentially) burn more calories for the same distance performed.

To be taken into account:

On a treadmill, the effort performed does not come from the legs, but from the treadmill. It is a cyclical turnover, which slightly favours the effort to be performed.

This can have some relevance for "moderate effort" sessions or during the supervision of a client with obesity for example.

Conclusion:

Apart from certain specific cases for a moderate effort or in the case of a disease… If the weather isn't bad, enjoy the beautiful weather!

63. Home training VS Gym training

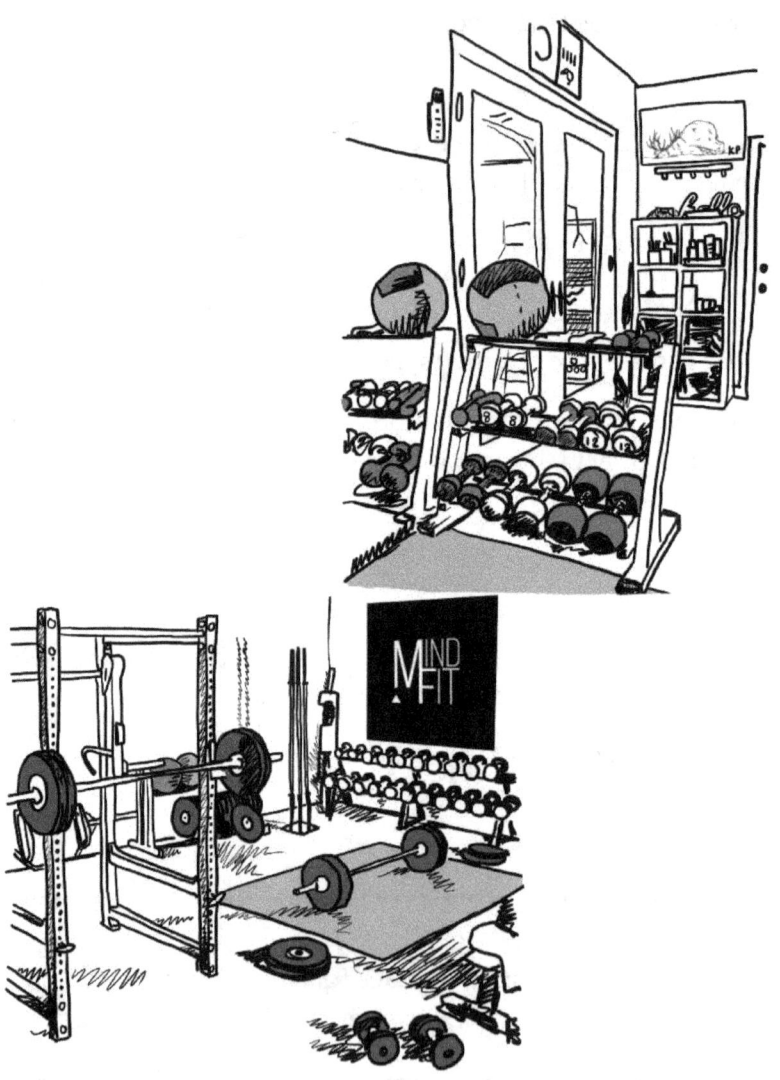

The goal is not to say that one is better than the other. Nonetheless, there are some points which can be interesting to take into account for a training at the gym or at home.

The advantages of training at the gym:

- Availability of a large choice of equipment

- Possibility to benefit from some advice given by coaches

- You have the possibility to make yourself spotted by someone or by a coach when you want to test your capacities on a movement with a heavy load

- The group effect. When you see others train, this can motivate you.

The disadvantages of training at the gym:

- You must organise your training times depending on the opening times of the gym

- The cost. We often forget that on top of the cost of the subscription, there is also the transportation cost to reach the gym. And we do not take into account the eventual annual indexations as well as the speeding fines if we are late on our planning!

- The time. Apart from the minutes that you spend in the gym for your training, there is the transportation time (round trip) to take into account. It might be productive time that is loft for something else!

- Although some advice is welcome, the Jean-Patrick which come speak to you about the last episode of their favourite TV show whilst you are in the midst of an effort... No thank you!

- The cleanliness of the gym.

- The unwanted closures of gyms. Be it because of a pandemic, construction works or other. It is not always wanted, but there are lost trainings!

- The monopolisation of the equipment

- The lack of intimacy (e.g. the sight of others)

The advantage of training at home:

- Time saving. No need to move from home! You have the possibility to save time on your day and be more productive during that one. This can also come with less stress.

- Financial gain. Regarding costs involving a regular frequency (e.g. monthly subscription), these will not be involved anymore! In certain cases, you do not lose money in fuel to go to the gym if you use a car.

- No one will disturb you.

- You can listen to the music you want. OK, there are headphones. But we have already all experienced finding ourselves with a low battery in the gym or simply forgetting our headphones/ headset. At home, no more problems!

- You can choose your fitness equipment. Contrarily to what we could think, there is no need to have equipment worth 30 000€ to train efficiently and have a long-term progression.

- You can also improve at home. Let's make it clear, overtime, you will need to invest in equipment to train at home. Nonetheless, having effective training methods will be required.

The disadvantages of training at home:

- Security: When you plan to use a heavy load, being spotted is not possible, unless you have a friend come over. You must be careful.

- Unless you are self-educated, learning will take more time that if you surround yourself.

- Lack of professionals to supervise you.

- Space. A room of 25-30m2 is ideal for a home gym, but not everyone benefits from that. You can train in a smaller space, hoping that you are not claustrophobic.

- The use of space. We don't all have the possibility to exploit the ground, the walls and/ or the ceiling to put a rack, rings or a storage area there (unless you are the owner or that you have the consent of the owner to do some renovation works as a tenant).

Motivation. Some struggle to find the motivation to train at home as they do not benefit from a unique room dedicated to training. In fact, training between the table of the living room and the kitchen is not convenient. Although I think the discipline component overpowers the motivational aspect (what should be done will be done; no matter how, no matter when and no matter where), it is obvious that training in space dedicated for physical activity is easier and more motivating that training in a room which is not dedicated for the practise of sports.

Conclusion:

There are advantages and disadvantages at the gym like at home.

Make the choice which suits you!

64. Machines VS Free weights

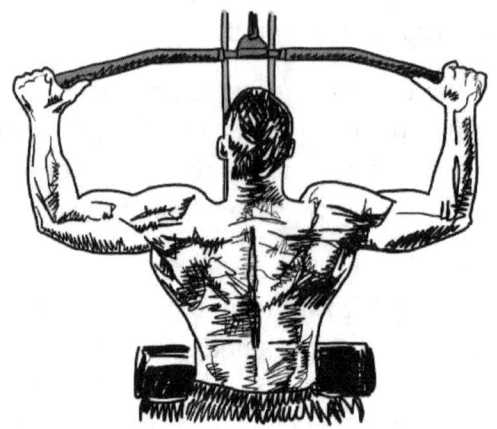

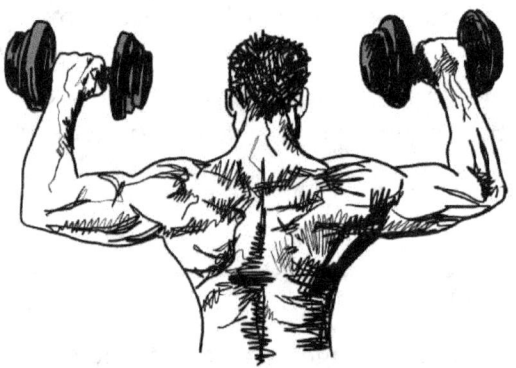

It is not to say that one type of work is better than the other depending on the equipment used. A machine totally has its place in training and it can be interesting in certain situations.

What are the potential advantages and disadvantages?[xcix]

It is what we will look at below:

- Machines allow isolating certain muscles since stabiliser muscles are less involved.

- Free weights allow a greater selection of exercises compared with machines (e.g. the execution of a "Man Maker" with dumbbells)

- Working with free weights improves coordination and balance by recruiting stabiliser muscles.

- Working with free weights allows working with a greater variety of angles on certain movements.

> Conclusion:
>
> Although machines allow isolating certain muscles, they impose a movement which might not seem natural for certain individuals. They nonetheless remain interesting depending on the goal.

65. Occlusion Training VS Classical Training

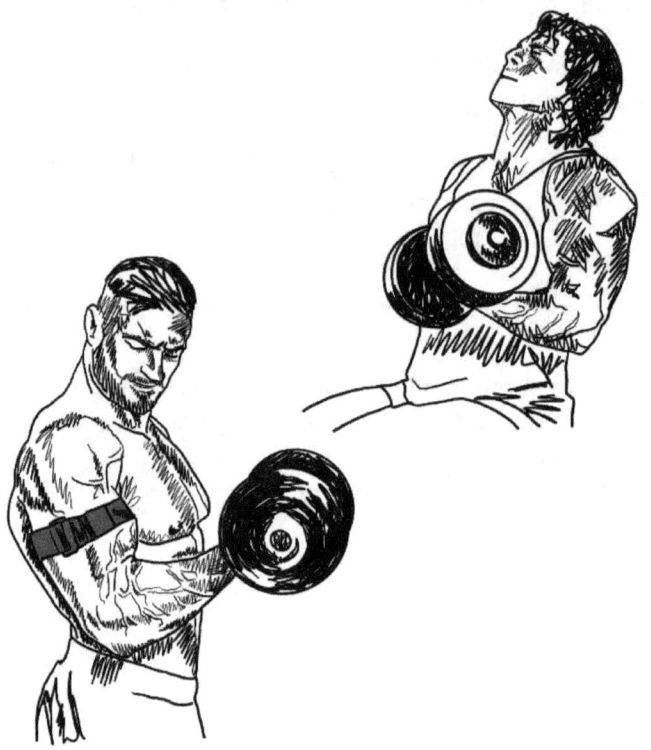

We already know what a classical training is. But occlusion training, that is another story!

Before comparing the two, here are a few explanations on occlusion training (but also on occlusion beyond training):

Occlusion training, also called B.F.R. (Blood Flow Restriction), involves cutting the venous blood flow of a limb, whilst allowing the arterial blood flow in a limb. This will allow generating "the pump"; in a nutshell, congestion. Occlusion training is performed by putting a strap or an elastic surrounding the limbs (arms or legs).

What does occlusion training bring compared to a classical training?

- Occlusion training favours hypertrophy with a lighter load than classical training (of course, the training programme plays an important role in the process).

- Occlusion training trains muscles and tendons.[ci] It can therefore be interesting to use it as a supplement to a main programme[cii]

- Strength gains from occlusion training are only observed in already trained individuals. For a beginner, it is therefore preferred to start with a "classical" training style rather than directly turning yourself to B.F.R.

- B.F.R. training allows reaching muscle failure more rapidly than a classical training with a similar load. This can be interesting to save time during sessions[ciii]

- Occlusion training can optimise your home trainings when you have little equipment

- Beyond training, occlusion work would allow to optimise recovery[civ]

To be taken into account:

There does not seem to be dangers linked with occlusion work when all the rules concerning that type of training are respected. If you have a doubt concerning its use or that you do not know how to use it, it is suggested to seek advice from a doctor or of a coach.

Conclusion:

Occlusion training can be an interesting supplement to your main training. In addition, that one can turn out being particularly effective following an injury to preserve your muscle gains or during deload phases in your training programme.

66. Overcoming Isometrics VS Yielding Isometrics

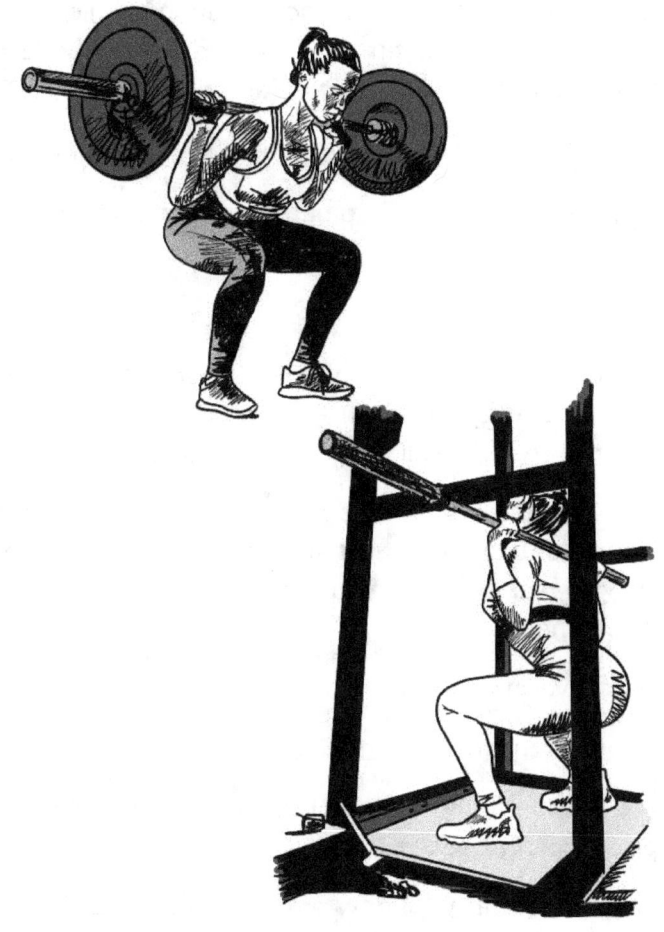

Here are interesting training methods! To understand these methods, it is important to understand the basics. Before speaking of Overcoming Isometrics and of Yielding Isometrics... We must first understand what isometry is and why it can be used, prior to speaking of methods linked to that one!

Isometrics:

Isometrics involve a contraction during which the insertion points of a muscle remain static and where the levers do not move, to resist to a fixed load (additional or gravity).[cv]

Examples of exercices: paused Back Squat, Plank, …

The advantages of the Isometrics contraction are multiple, here are a few[cvi]:

- Value for hypertrophy

- From 1 to 2 seconds of isometrics work, there is a limitation of elastic energy to produce in the concentric phase. There is therefore some value for the starting force.

- The strength gain is specific to the angle trained (It is important to consider that isometrics work at a long muscle length seems to benefit from a better transfer on the movement's whole range of motion)

- Improves mobility

<u>To be taken into account:</u>

We consider that there is a loss of strength of 5 to 10% for each pre-concentric second[73] above 2 seconds.

Well. Now that we know more about isometrics training, we can now compare both methods related to this type of work. That is, Overcoming Isometrics and Yielding Isometrics.

---

[73] Before the concentric phase of a movement

Overcoming Isometrics:[cvii]

It consists of pushing a light load (e.g. unloaded barbell) against a resistance which cannot move (e.g. pushing an unloaded Olympic barbell on a Back Squat against a rack). The goal here is to push as strongly as possible depending on your capacities (putting a maximal speed intention). The principal advantage of this method would be a strength gain on the trained angle whilst allowing for a large recruitment of muscle fibres on the concentric phase. This method also has a value for athletes in-season as it would allow preserving our strength without creating too much muscular fatigue which could harm the practice of sports. It also proves to be interesting in a process of rehabilitation.

Yielding Isometrics:[cviii]

Contrarily to overcoming isometrics, this type of isometrics is performed on the eccentric phase of the movement. The goal of this method is to bring a strength gain (on the eccentric phase), to improve the health of connective tissues, to improve deceleration capacities, it can be be used for athletes' rehabilitation and for hypertrophy. It is possible to go to failure with this method and it can be used with or without equipment depending on the planification and on the goal of the supervised athlete. On the mental side, this method would allow optimising the motivational factor of the athlete because it represents a real physical challenge. When it is well used and that all the factors of training are taken into account (intensity, time under tension, loads used…), it would also allow improving the capacity to recruit and to synchronise motor units (intramuscular coordination) even in dynamic movements.

> Conclusion:
>
> The two isometrics methods can be used in trainings to gain or to maintain strength. This will depend on your goals and on the individualisation of your programme.

67. Dumbbells VS Kettlebells

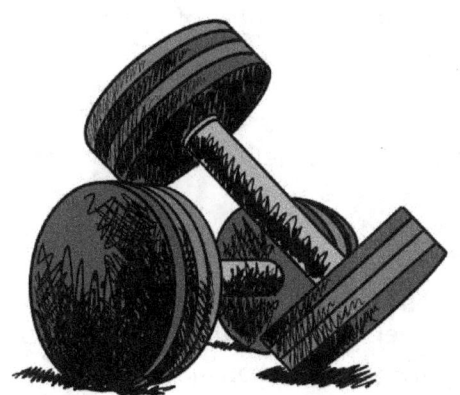

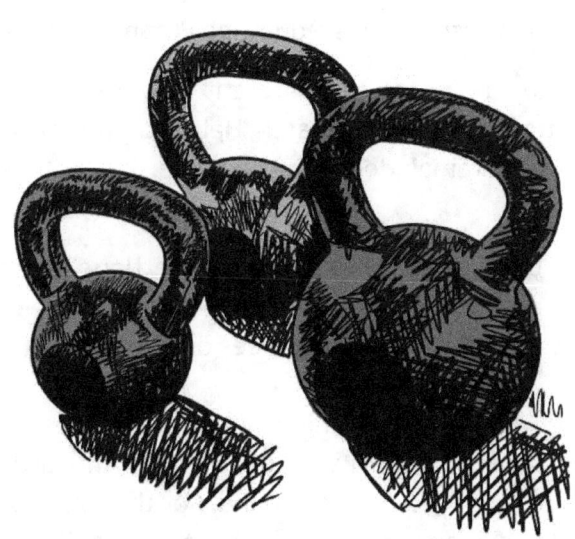

A topic[cix] already examined in the fitness world, but it is always good to understand why choosing certain equipment depending on your goals. Let's go for the comparison!

- According to its geometry, the kettlebell has nothing to do with a dumbbell. The strengths' centre of application is far from its axis of rotation.

- Compared to a dumbbell, the Kettlebell is the most compact tool.

- Unlike a dumbbell (and depending on the tool's position relative to the arm), when we grab the kettlebell (by the handle), its centre of gravity is found outside of the hand.

- It is easier to use a dumbbell than a kettlebell.

Depending on the different movements typical to kettlebells trainings (Swing, Snatch, Half-Snatch, Clean & Long Cycle), here is the remainder of the analyses:

- Due to its compactness, a Kettlebell, and even two, easily passes in between the legs[74], there were a dumbbell would risk hitting the legs, the knees or the thighs.

- Always, during this circular arc movement, the Kettlebell's centre of gravity is located 10-15cm farther away from the elbow than from the hand. For the same execution speed, the necessary strength to control the Kettlebell will be even greater. This even more so increases the effect of the exercise.

---

[74] This will depend on your morpho-anatomy and on the Kettlebell model used

Conclusion:

The kettlebell is a tool which is more versatile than the dumbbell, but which requires more mastery to know how to use it correctly contrarily to a dumbbell. We must not neglect a tool at the expense of another, but rather know when and how to use it.

68. Triceps Extension (bar) : Pronated VS supinated

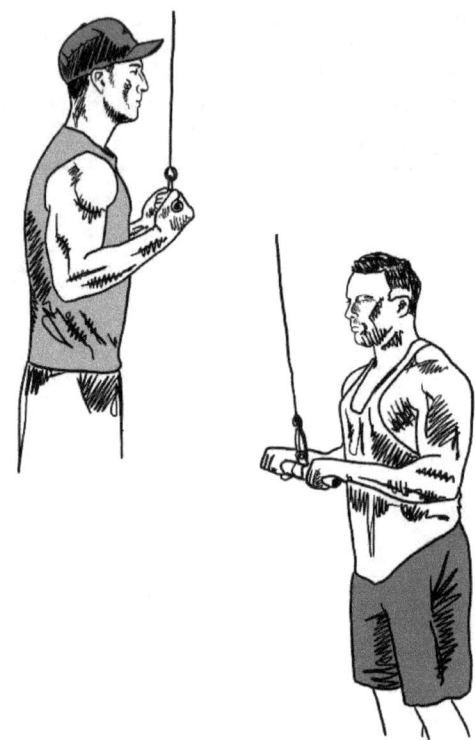

Before knowing whether there is a value to alternating the grip for triceps' recruitment, we must understand which exercise we are talking about.

Although alternatives exist, we will not linger on the alternatives to this exercise, but on the work of the triceps' extension with a straight bar depending on the grip used.

It therefore goes without saying that we are not talking of an extension performed with a neutral grip (e.g. the rope).

So, is there are a real value between the pronated and the supinated grips on that exercise? Let's take a closer look!

To correctly perform the "triceps extension" exercise, we are meant to keep the arms aligned with the forearms to limit the risk of injuries.

According to certain individuals, the supinated grip would allow accentuating the work on the triceps. The movement is often harder to execute due to the grip of the bar (forearms) and due to the fact that it is hard to completely extend our arms at the end of the movement (principally due to the wrists' mobility).

When we lack mobility, the pronated grip allows a better elbow extension than the pronated grip on a straight bar[cx]. This potentially leads to better muscle gains. In addition, the force exerted by the forearms is reduced on this exercise with the straight bar.

From an anatomical standpoint, the triceps (muscle) is not attached to the radius (bone) but to the ulna (bone). This means that wanting to pass from a pronated grip to a supinated grip on the grounds that we would better work a portion of the muscle makes no sense because the muscular recruitment of the triceps is not influenced by changing the grip position.[cxi]

The only thing to memorise concerning the supinated grip on the triceps extension exercise performed with a straight bar is that it does not allow a better muscle activation on the triceps compared to a pronated grip.

Conclusion:

On the Triceps extension exercise, there is absolutely no value in using the supinated grip.

69. American Swing VS Russian Swing

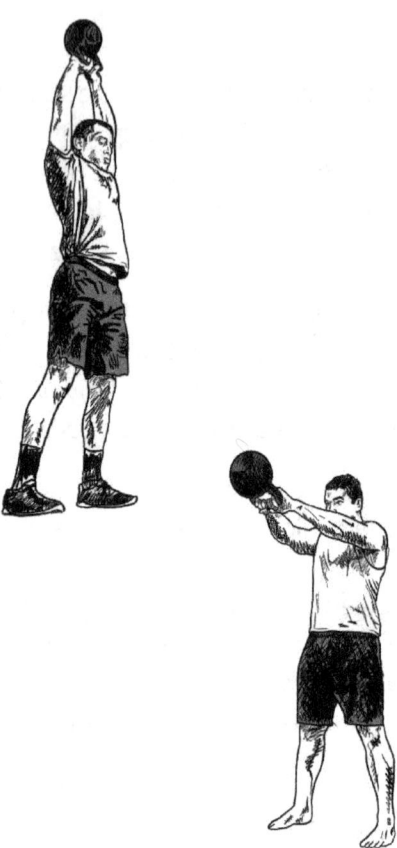

Before getting to the heart of the matter, it is important to know that the terms "Russian Swing" and "American Swing" are used for commercial purposes. A swing is a swing and there is not one single way to do some kettlebell swing. It is an exercise which is adaptable to the majority of individuals. And after having had multiple exchanges with Stéphane Dogman[75], my opinion converges with his on the fact that the swing can also be modified depending on the targeted goal.

---

[75] Cfr: article 8

Here are a few explanations which will allow seeing things more clearly:

-       The Russian Swing allows carrying a heavier load than the American Swing.

-       The Russian Swing allows performing more repetitions than the American Swing during a given time.

-       In the case of a kyphosis and by adapting the height of the kettlebell during the ballistic movement, the Russian Swing can be interesting to continue working the extension of the hip and of the posterior chain comparatively to an American Swing which can turn out to be dangerous.

-       The Russian Swing can be interesting for the practice of powerlifting and to have a certain transfer on the Deadlift. Here where American Swing will certainly be less interesting.

-       The American Swing can have a transfer for weightlifting by favouring the triple extension (ankle – knee – hip). Nonetheless, the movement will be more vertical, which will neglect the initially planned work with the swing.

Conclusion:

Unless you are performing CrossFit for competitive purposes where we can find this movement, there is no value in using the American Swing.

70. Front Pulldown vs Behind The Neck Pulldown

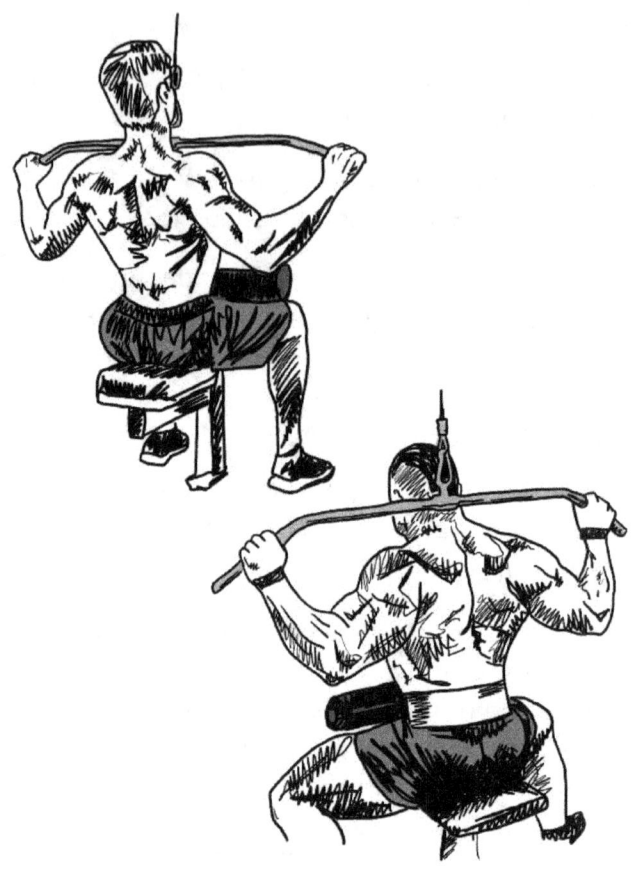

Let's directly get to the heart of the topic by analysing both movements:

-   There is little value in practising Behind the Neck Pulldown in terms of muscle recruitment since the latissimus dorsi will be significantly more recruited during a pull movement where the bar comes in front of the head.[cxii]

- The position of the Behind the Neck Pulldown generally places the arms in an important horizontal abduction, which requires a good shoulder and scapula mobility. It is why this movement is often criticised in weight training. It would imply more risks of injury on an articular level (glenohumeral joint and cervical).

- The Behind the Neck Pulldown seems to not bring any additional benefits in terms of muscle involvement compared with the Neck Pulldown.

- What corresponds to the Neck Pulldown in terms of transfer is similar to Pull Ups. In addition, it is not an easily transferable movement in a discipline or in everyday life.

To be taken into account:

Maybe have you already heard that this movement is "dangerous" due to the shape of the acromion which can cause trouble with adjacent structures. I have a nuanced opinion on that problematic. It is the lack of lucidity on the progression which is dangerous. In addition, it is difficult to know the shape of our acromion and it is not because we practise this movement that we will necessarily injure ourselves. During a discussion, a coach and a rehabilitation trainer explained to me that the adjacent structures are already in contact with the acromion, with the subacromial bursa and that all the ligaments are only the prolongation of the joint capsule. According to him, the idea of the subacromial conflict is erroneous. It is a viewpoint that I share. Everything is to be nuanced.

> Conclusion:
>
> The trend seems to put forward the Behind the Neck Pulldown as an uninteresting exercise for your programme as it brings no value compared with the Front Pulldown concerning hypertrophy. Caution would say we must remain agnostic and that in a well-defined context, this one could still have a value. What matters is to know why to use it.

PART 4: FOR OR AGAINST?

"For how many spirits thinking is not weighing the pros and the cons, but inclining towards something!" [Pierre Baillargeon]

71. The protective foam pad: for or against?

FOR!

Nonetheless, my point of view will differ according to the use of the foam pad depending on the exercise to be performed.

For the Zercher Squat? I am for! When we do not have elbow pads, this can remove the inconvenience caused in the crook of the elbow for the practice of the exercise.

For the Hip Thrust? I am for!

The use of a foam pad is useful, almost mandatory to avoid feeling pain on the hips and knowing how to work securely and without discomfort.

For the Back Squat? I am against (or at least, not particularly for)!

Often used because it hurts the back of the neck, it can bring another problem by unbalancing the barbell[76]. By unbalancing the barbell, this can modify the movement in a bad way (deterioration of the technical gesture).

The first thing to do if we want to do some Back Squat, and mostly, execute the movement well, would be to learn to correctly engage the back muscles, and more specifically the trapezius muscles if we perform a "High Bar" Squat (barbell located above the trapezius muscles). If we do not feel comfortable with the "High Bar", the "Low Bar" (barbell located below the trapezius muscles) in a Back Squat movement can have its stake, but the movement will differ slightly (it can also be more restrictive from a mobility standpoint for some).

---

[76] Back Squat: here we are referring to an Olympic bar squat. The safety bar is not involved.

Certain people or coaches will favour the use of the protection foam pad in the case of an injury on the Back Squat. Personally, I do not share this opinion. I find that some alternatives are more interesting in the case of an injury, like changing exercise or using another equipment for example.

Conclusion:

I am not against the foam pad. I am just against its use in certain situations as it can bring more drawbacks than benefits.

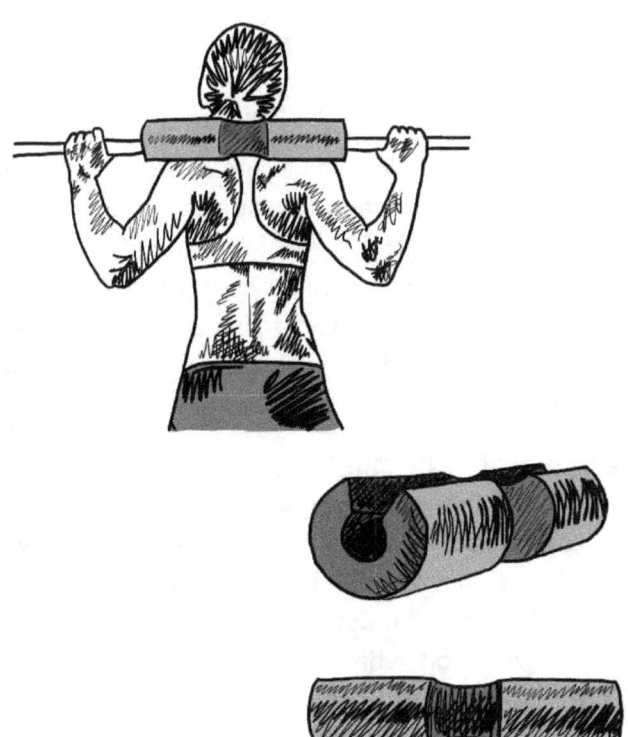

72. Arnold Press: For or against?

I am not particularly against even though I don't use it anymore (that will perhaps change one day) in my training programmes. And yet, I love Arnold Schwarzenegger!

The Arnold Press, I've done, and I've done again a lot of it since I originally like this exercise. But, for many reasons, I do not use it anymore.

The first one being that we carry lighter loads on the Arnold Press compared with the "classic" dumbbells Shoulder Press (all by keeping a certain similarity between the movements). This does not mean that I found the Arnold Press useless. It is an observation that I am doing because, according to me, the strength of an individual is key to his health and for his progress.

The second reason principally involves the injury risk on the rotator cuff. In fact, performing a rotation movement with two dumbbells in each hand is demanding, especially when that one asks for a rotation during the course of the movement. I still want to temper my words considering that tissues adapt themselves depending on the mechanical constraint they go through. Overtime, muscle, bone and collagen tissues become more resilient and resistant.

The third, and probably the most important, is the mastery of the basics. This is only my opinion, but I do not consider the Arnold Press to be a core movement with a goal of muscle gain. With regards to "pressing" movements to the shoulders. The standing Shoulder Press must first be mastered before considering any variation whatsoever. And if your mobility allows it, perform a standing Shoulder Press with dumbbells.

Alternatives to the Arnold Press which can have some value in specific cases of course exist, but this relates to a specific public with an intermediate, or even with an advanced level.

Conclusion:

I do not consider the Arnold Press useless but it is not a priority in a training programme according to me.

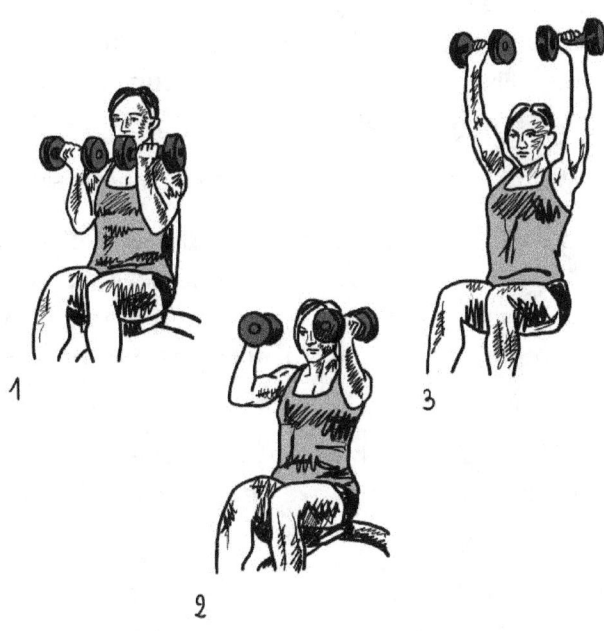

73. Squeeze Press (Plate) / Close grip Bench Press (with plates): For or against?

AGAINST!

According to me, this exercise is a waste of time and is completely useless.

This exercise is similar to a dumbbell Bench Press, except that rather than holding dumbbells from either side of the hand, we will take a plate by pressing with the flat of the hands on the plate and carrying the load from top-down, like on a traditional Bench Press. Finally, according to the popular belief this would effectively work the middle chest.

Let's now look at why I find this exercise completely useless:

- This exercise is not ergonomic. This is subjective, I give you that. But taking a plate, setting ourselves on the bench, squeezing it with all our strength without letting it move and doing our repetitions... It is not the most convenient way to perform an exercise!

- It is impossible to measure the power of the pressure exerted on the plate for the average individual. This means we cannot measure a notable progression on that exercise.

- We are limited in terms of range of motion. This is bothering since, originally, movements which resemble the Bench Press have the goal of having an important stretching tension.

- We are limited by the load. In fact, not many gyms propose plates of 30, 40 or 50kg.

- The Squeeze Press does not work the middle chest. From an anatomical standpoint, the chest is composed of three heads. The clavicular head, the sternal head and the abdominal head. This means that there is nothing in the middle of our chest. And we cannot change the shape of a muscle.

> Conclusion:
>
> The Squeeze Press does not work the middle chest and it does not bring real advantages to your muscle hypertrophy.

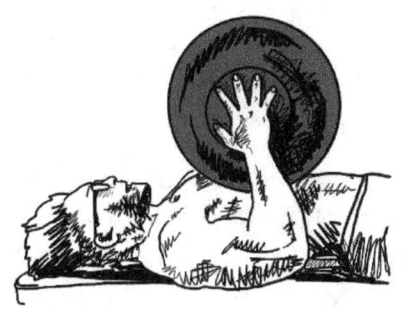

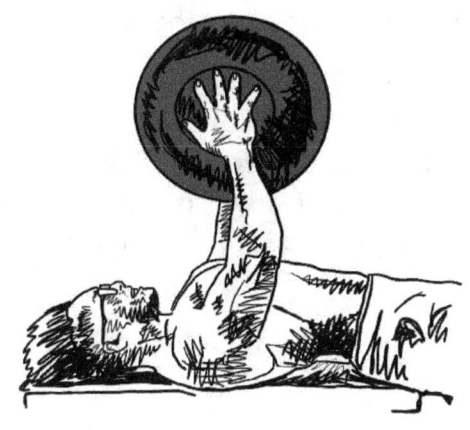

74. Shrug Rotation: For or against?

AGAINST!

I am not against shrugs. They have their value, according to me, in weightlifting for example. However, it is the rotation which I see as particularly useless for the development of the trapezius.

Shrugs with rotation[77] are principally used with dumbbells and they involve shrugging your shoulders and then doing a rearward rotation movement (some even practise it forwards) to go back to their initial place before following up with new repetitions.

The first reason why I don't hold Shrugs with a rotation close to my heart is that it could negatively influence the health of your shoulders.[cxiii] I insist on the "could" since I remain nuanced on the topic knowing that, initially, I think that no movement is fundamentally bad. Tissues adapt depending on the mechanical constraint they endure[78].

The second reason is that the rotational movement does not allow a sufficient tension to recruit the medial trapezius after having put a sufficient tension on the upper trapezius. It would be more interesting to lean the torso to obtain a sufficient tension on these ones whilst avoiding rotations.

---

[77] Shrug with rotation: Popularised by Kevin Levron, a North-American bodybuilder of the 90's era

[78] Already mentioned in the theme "Arnold Press: For or against?"

Better ways exist to effectively recruit the trapezius muscles. Of course, it all depends on the context. But some exercises like Y elevations or the "Face Pull" are good alternatives for the recruitment of your trapezius muscles when these ones are well executed.

To be taken into account:

If you want to use the Shrug to develop the upper part of your trapezius, there is the possibility to optimise their recruitment by doing a slight 30 degrees abduction of the arm when you use dumbbells (or kettlebells). In fact, a study[cxiv] demonstrated that the results were significantly superior in terms of muscular activation when a slight shoulder abduction was applied.

The results are very interesting for individuals practising weight training which are looking to maximise their muscle hypertrophy gains towards the upper trapezius muscles. A wider grip would therefore be recommended. The protocol presented here involves the use of dumbbells (and an intensity of 25% MVIC – Maximum voluntary isometric contraction); the 30-degree abduction generated from the start of the movement thus implies an additional activation which will have to be maintained throughout the whole movement. Yet, with a heavy load (> 70% 1RM – Magnetic Resonance Imaging), this abduction will be very difficult to maintain. Hence, a wide grip with a bar could perhaps resolve that problem.[cxv]

Conclusion:

The rotation on the Shrug exercise does not present any value.

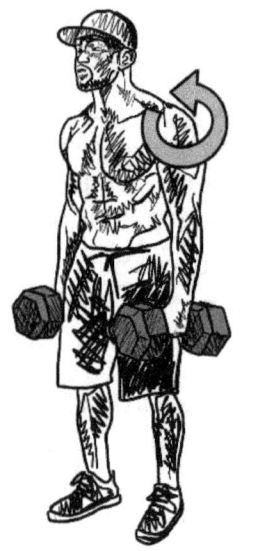 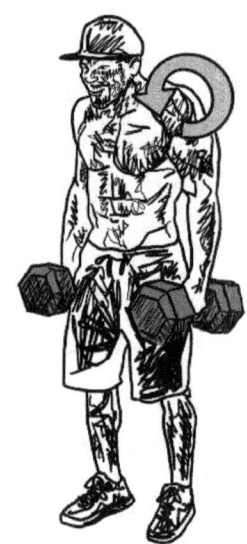

75. Behind The Neck Press: For or against?

FOR!

This exercise has long been criticised for being dangerous and for not bringing any benefits to obtain notable muscle gains.

It is clear that I would not put the Behind The Neck Press in the session's main body[79], and even less as a core exercise if I had the goal of shoulder hypertrophy.

Nonetheless, I think that it can prove itself interesting in a warm up. And here are the advantages that the Behind The Neck Press can bring if it is well executed: This allows fighting against eventual imbalances of the internal rotators.

- Recruitment of the shoulder external rotators. This allows fighting against eventual imbalances of the internal rotators.

- Fight against a sedentary position and against kyphosis[80].

- Allows involving certain muscles which stabilise the scapula, which can contribute to an interesting transfer on certain exercises (e.g.: Bench Press).

But how to execute it correctly?

If the Behind The Neck Press can turn out to be advantageous in certain situations, it goes without saying that its execution must be exemplary. Certain aspects will therefore have to be taken into account for the starting position:

---

[79]   The session's body: middle of the session

[80]   Kyphosis: Deviation of the spine which renders the back convex (Definition of the French Robert Dictionary)

- The grip width slightly larger than shoulder width

- The elbows must be placed under the bar (recruitment of the external rotators)

- Fixing the scapula and keeping it in a depressed position

- Keeping the pelvis neutral

To be taken into account:

Some people struggle maintaining the position as they accumulate repetitions. In fact, this can modify the recruitment of motor units and once again enable the internal rotators dominate. This can also be explained by a lack of mobility. We can suggest not lowering as much and limiting ourselves at the occiput (the back of the skull) to keep the external rotators engaged as the repetitions progress.

Conclusion:

The Behind The Neck Press can be useful to fight against postural disequilibrium (shoulders forward).

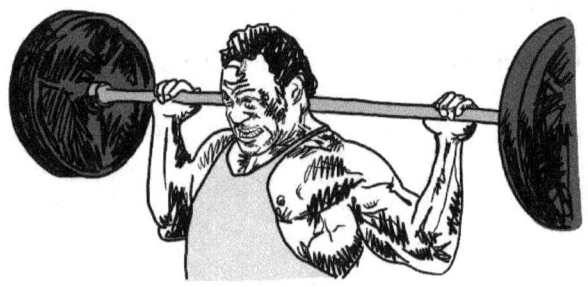

76. Bench Press Suicide Grip: For or against?

AGAINST!

This exercise is similar to the Bench Press in all ways except that the grip differs since the thumb does not surround the bar. In fact, all the fingers are on the same side to that one.

Why use it?

According to certain athletes, this would help optimising their performance and would allow them having a better position, or at least, be more comfortable during the exercise.

Nonetheless, I always take into account the risk-benefit factor in a programme. That is why I am against.

The suicide grip, which we also call the "false grip" or even the "Thumbless grip", is suicidal, as its name indicates.

It is not possible to take the bar in a straight manner with the suicide grip. The wrists will automatically be "bent". It is therefore not possible to keep the bar in neutral position. This can be painful for some people. In addition, the bar risks sliding and so falling onto you. This constitutes a danger.

If you really desire to continue using the suicide grip after what I've just stated, it is then better practising it on a Smith machine for more security, or with a spotter (someone which secures you during the entire lift's duration).

Conclusion:

The "suicide grip" brings more risks than it does benefits on the Bench Press.

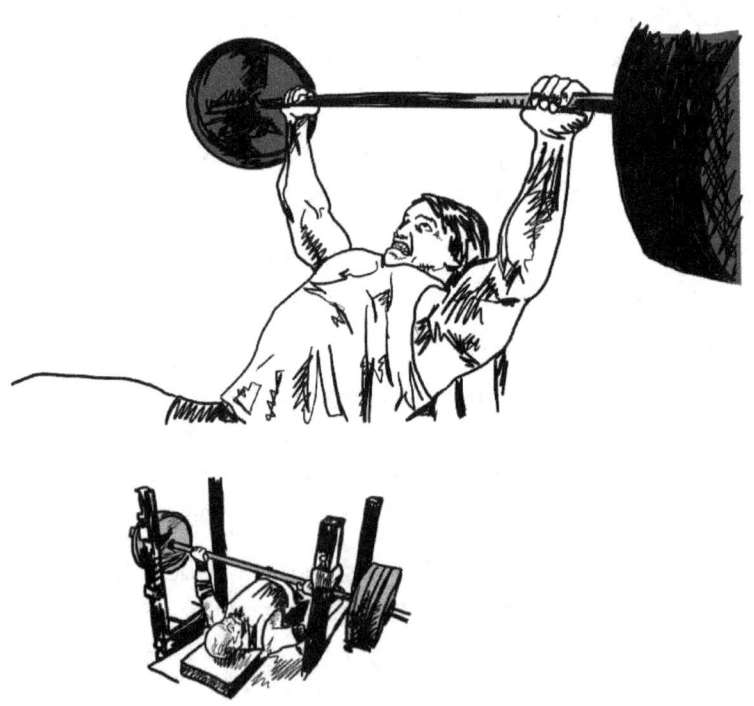

77. Weight plate Side Bend: For or against?

AGAINST! (Well, that seems a bit radical. Rather, let's say that I don't see much value in it!)

In any case, with a muscle growth goal and with a plate (for the spine's health, it is another story).

You've probably already seen it in a gym or on social media. This exercise has for goal to target the oblique muscles by inclining yourself on the sides with the help of a plate.

The idea makes sense. So, why don't I recommend it?

For the simple and good reason that this exercise does not bring enough intensity. Especially in the case where you use a plate. The plate is already an important limitation in terms of load (although plates of above 25kg do exist).

One of the most important factors for muscle development... Is intensity.

When you realise 35 repetitions or more and that this does not prevent you from "easily" continuing your set (that is, by being far from muscular failure), it is that the intensity is simply not high enough.

In addition, depending on your level, there is little doubt that the grip (hands, fingers and forearms) will let go before your oblique muscles do.

Finally, and that is often where the problem is found, the execution of the movement is far too often neglected.

It would be more interesting to include an alternative if you really want to work your oblique muscles, such as the exercise: "Wood Chopper" on the cable machine which would allow putting a greater intensity as well as a greater range of motion.

> Conclusion:
>
> The abdominal incline with a plate to engage your oblique muscles does not come with enough intensity to bring a notable progress when muscle growth is the goal. Nonetheless, take into consideration that the plate is only the tool. The "side bend" is totally viable as an exercise if we have the capacity of increasing the load.

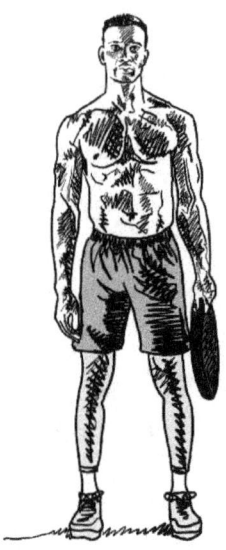
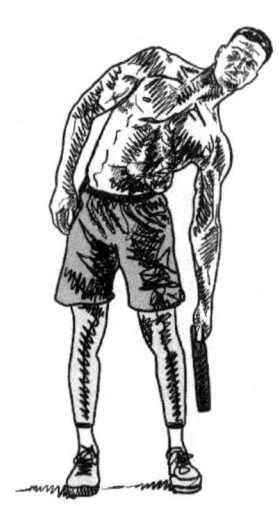

Acknowledgments

I would like to, very particularly, thank the people who have contributed to the creation of this publication, and more particularly:

Mathilde Schmitt, translator of the French version to the English version that you have just read.

Kelig Pinson, illustrator, for the drawings realised and for her numerous hours of work which allow better understanding the publication.

Ghaïs Guelaïa, for sharing his knowledge as well as for the reading of, and the corrections brought to, the initial text in French.

Alka Matewa, professionnl Muay thaï fighter and actor, for having accepted to be illustrated in this book.

My family and my friends, for the support they gave me for this life project

Every one which has not been cited in this section of acknowledgments and which have contributed to the creation of this book.

About the author...

Nicolas Genotte is born on the 9th of November 1993 in Marche-en-Famenne in Belgium.

Since his youngest age, he is an all-rounder as it relates to sports (judo, waterpolo, running, basketball, …)

It is therefore naturally that he orients himself towards a "sport study" ("sport étude" in French) cursus at the "Athénée royal Liège Atlas", prior to directing himself towards a bachelor of "specialised educator in socio-sporting" ("bachelier d'éducateur spécialisé en activités socio-sportives" in French) at the "Haute École Parnasse-ISEI". At 21 years old, freshly graduated, he started his career of sports coach in 2015 by pursuing certifications every year with the goal of professionalising himself in this profession.

In 2017, then 23 years of age, he founds MindFit BXL, an association of sports and healthcare professionals. The latter has for goal to provide the best possible support the clients during a sports coaching in order to be the best prepared to all sorts of problematics. He is also the co-founder of the online course centre CF2S of which the goal is to encourage coaches, physiotherapists and athletes to continue learning and updating their knowledge overtime as it relates to health and fitness professions.

Via his work as a programmer in his fields, he also managed to bring multiple kettlebell sport athletes to an elite level.

He also does programmes for weight training Brazilian jiujitsu, motorcross & surf athletes.

He also possesses a YouTube Channel called "MindFit BXL" of which the goal is to keep informed and improve the knowledge of people wishing to take care of their health. He makes informative vignettes and he invites guests qualified within the domains of sport, health and nutrition.

As an athlete...

It is only by the age of 21 years old that Nicolas starts to interest himself to the kettlebell, and to the development of strength and to different training methods by starting CrossFit. It is only 3 years later that he decides specialising himself on the use of the kettlebell and participating to his first international competition as an amateur.

After, everything goes very fast. A few months later, Nicolas Genotte becomes the first Belgian of history to reach the elite status in the IKMF federation (International Kettlebell Marathon Federation & associated disciplines) and to qualify for the world championships.

In November 2018 in Spain, Nicolas Genotte ended double Bronze medalist in Elite division in Light Weight category. A grand premiere for a young 24 years old athlete which had only started competing 9 months earlier.

A promising start of career which led to the title of world champion in Poland in 2019 and a European title in 2021, as well as the award of "honorific title of Master of Sport" ("titre honorifique" in French) by the president of the federation.

Nicolas Genotte is also passionate about other sports which target the development of strength, but not only. He opens up to several sports disciplines and, above all, he wants to make kettlebell sport more known in Belgium in order for that one to be recognised by the general public.

REFERENCING:

[i] The Pelvis & Low Back relationship, Squat University, 2017 [ii] One Of the Squat's Most Controversial Questions Answered, Aaron Lipsey, 2013

[iii] "Le Butt Wink", Olivier Bolliet, 2020

[iv] Flexion lombaire présente chez powerlifters qui font du deadlift ou squat (thèse), Edington 2017

Ce que tu ne sais pas sur le dos rond, Alexis Beck, 2 mai 2022, IG

Porter dos rond : et si ça avait du bon ? Ce que disent les études scientifiques., Les chroniques de la douleur, 2022, YT

[v] Anabolic steroid use in weightlifters and bodybuilders: an internet survey of drug utilization, Paul J. Perry & al, Clin J. Sport Med., 2005 [vi] « Pourquoi soulever lourd ? », Wikifit – outil d'entraînement [vii] Syllabus « Psychologie du sport », bachelier éducateur spécialisé en activités socio-sportives, Parnasse-ISEI, 2014

[viii] Hypertrophied cruciate ligament in high performance weightlifters observed in magnetic resonance imaging, Piotr Grzelak, corresponding author Michał Podgorski, Ludomir Stefanczyk, Marek Krochmalski, and Marcin Domzalski, 2012

Analysis of the load on the knee joint and vertebral column with changes in squatting depth and weight load, Hagen Hartmann 1, Klaus Wirth, Markus Klusemann, Sports Med., 2013

[ix] Associations between activities and LBP in adolescents, Astrid Noreng Sjolie, 2005

[x] Which physical activities and sports can be recommended to chronic low back pain patients after rehabilitation? A Ribaud 1, I Tavares, E Viollet, M Julia, C Hérisson, A Dupeyron, 2013

[xi] The Human Muscle Size and Strength Relationship: Effects of Architecture, Muscle Force, and Measurement Location, Balshaw & al., Medicine & Science in Sports & Exercise, 2021

[xii] Is there any non-functional training ? A conceptual review, Bernardo N. & al, 2022

Et si on arrêtait de parler d'entraînement « fonctionnel » ?, Clement Naveilhan, 18 janvier 2022, IG

[xiii] Effects of Strength Training on Running Economy in Highly Trained Runners: A Systematic Review with Meta-Analysis of Controlled Trials,
Balsalobre-Fernández, Carlos1; Santos-Concejero, Jordan2; Grivas, Gerasimos V., 2016

[xiv] Effects of different intensities of resistance exercise on regulators of myogenesis, Colin D Wilborn, 2009

[xv] Schoenfeld BJ, Grgic J, Ogborn D, Krieger JW. Strength and Hypertrophy Adaptations Between Low- vs. High-Load Resistance Training: A Systematic Review and Meta-analysis. J Strength Cond Res. 2017 Dec;31(12):3508-3523 4.Goto K, Ishii N, Kizuka T, Takamatsu K.

The impact of metabolic stress on hormonal responses and muscular adaptations. Med Sci Sports Exerc. 2005 Jun;37(6):955-63.

Carroll KM, Bazyler CD, Bernards JR, Taber CB, Stuart CA, DeWeese BH, Sato K, Stone MH. Skeletal Muscle Fiber Adaptations Following Resistance Training Using Repetition Maximums or Relative Intensity. Sports (Basel). 2019 Jul 11

Goldberg AL, Etlinger JD, Goldspink DF, Jablecki C. Mechanism of work-induced hypertrophy of skeletal muscle. Med Sci Sports. 1975 Fall

Effect of repetitions duration during resistance training on muscle hypertrophy : a systematic review and meta-analysis

Piazzesi G, Reconditi M, Linari M, Lucii L, Bianco P, Brunello E, Decostre V, Stewart A, Gore DB, Irving TC, Irving M, Lombardi V. Skeletal muscle performance determined by modulation of number of myosin motors rather than motor force or stroke size. Cell. 2007 Nov

Set volume for muscle site : The Ultimate evidence based bible – Weightology

High Resistance-Training Volume Enhances Muscle Thickness in Resistance-Trained Men. Brigatto et al. (2019).

[xvi] gh-Intensity Intermittent Exercise and Fat Loss, https://www.researchgate.net/profile/SteveSteve Boutcher, 2010-2011

[xvii] Total Daily energy expenditure is increased following a single bout of sprint interval training, Kyle J. Sevits & al, 2013

Two minuts of sprint-interval exercise elicits 24hr oxygen consumption similar to that of 30min of continuous endurance exercise, Tom J Hazell & al, 2012

Slow and steady or hard and fast ? A systematic review and metaanalysis of studies comparing body composition changes between interval training and moderate intensity continuous training, James Steele & al., 2021

[xviii] Magnitude and duration of excess of post-exercise oxygen consumption between high-intensity interval and moderate-intensity continuous exercise: A systematic review. Obesity Reviews., Panissa V. & al., 2021

[xix] Br J. Sport Med, O'sullivan, 2012

[xx] Resistance training vs. static stretching: effects on flexibility and strength, Sam K Morton 1, James R Whitehead, Ronald H Brinkert, Dennis J Caine, 2011

[xxi] The Interactions of Intensity, Frequency and Duration of Exercise Training in Altering Cardiorespiratory Fitness, Howard A. Wenger, 2012

[xxii] Relationships Between Anthropometry and Maximal Strength in Male Classic Powerlifters, Pierre-Marc Ferland, Antoine Laurier, Alain Steve Comtois, PubMed, 2020

xxiii   Effect of ankle mobility and segment ratios on trunk lean in the barbell back squat, Emil L. Fuglsang, Anders S. Telling, Henrik Sorensen, 2017

xxiv   Squat très incliné : longs fémurs ou manque de mobilité ? Charlotte Vedel, 7 septembre 2021, IG

xxv   Impact of range of motion during ecologically valid resistance training protocols on muscle size, subcutaneous fat and strength, Gerard E McMahon, Christopher I Morse, Adrian Burden, Keith Winwood, Gladys L Onambélé, 2014

L'amplitude au développé couché : comment la choisir selon ses objectifs ? Geek'n'fit, 24 avril 2021, IG

xxvi   Analyse Event 4 1000m row Reebok CrossFit Games 2020, Sport Sciences Therapist, 30 octobre 2020, IG

xxvii   Article de rédaction L'haltérophilie chez le jeune : attention danger

[xxix] Resistance training among young athletes: safety, efficacy and injury prevention effects, A D Faigenbaum1 and G D Myer, 2009 [xxx] Schumann et al. (2022) : "Compatibility of Concurrent Aerobic and Strength Training for Skeletal Muscle Size and Function : An Updated Systematic Review and Meta-Analysis"

Wilson et al. (2012) : "Concurrent Training: A Meta-Analysis Examining Interference of Aerobic and Resistance Exercises

Fyfe et al. (2014) : "Interference between Concurrent Resistance and Endurance Exercise : Molecular Bases and the Role of Individual Training Variables

L'effet d'interférence : Le cardio peut-il nuire à la prise de muscle ? Gael Lemaitre, 2022, IG

A proposed model for examining the interference phenomenon between concurrent aerobic and strength training, Docherty, 2000

Concurrent strength and endurance training. A review, Leveritt & al., 1999

The acute effects of strength, endurance and concurrent exercises on the Akt/mTOR/p70S6K1 and AMPK signaling pathway responses in rat skeletal muscle, De Souza & al, 2013

[xxxi] The nature and prevalence of injury during CrossFit training, Paul Taro Hak 1, Emil Hodzovic, Ben Hickey, 2013

[xxxii] The Benefits and Risks of CrossFit: A Systematic Review, Jena Meyer, Janet Morrison, Julie Zuniga, 2017

Sciences du sport : Fréquence et nature des blessures en CrossFit, P. Debraux, 2013

[xxxiii] Injury Incidence and Patterns Among Dutch CrossFit Athletes, Mirwais Mehrab, Robert-Jan de Vos, Gerald A Kraan, Nina M C Mathijssen, 2017

Sciences du Sport : Bénéfices et risques du CrossFit, A. Manolova, 2018

[xxxiv] Définition « Muscle Memory, Wiki.

[xxxv] The Impact of Endurance Training on Human Skeletal Muscle Memory, Global Isoform Expression and Novel Transcripts, Maléne E Lindholm, Stefania Giacomello, Beata Werne Solnestam, Helene Fischer, Mikael Huss, Sanela Kjellqvist, Carl Johan Sundberg, 2016

FuturaSanté, Marie-Céline Ray, 2016

[xxxvi] Resistance Training-Induced Elevations in Muscular Strength in Trained Men Are Maintained After 2 Weeks of Detraining and Not Differentially Affected by Whey Protein Supplementation, Paul S Hwang, Thomas L Andre, Sarah K McKinley-Barnard, Flor E Morales Marroquín, Joshua J Gann, Joon J Song, Darryn S Willoughby, 2017, J. Strength Cond Res.

[xxxvii] Evidence-Based Resistance Training Recommendations for Muscular Hypertrophy, J. Fisher, J. Steele, D. Smith, 2013, ResearchGate

[xxxviii] Cardiorespiratory and metabolic characteristics of detraining in humans, I Mujika, S Padilla, Med. Sci. Sports Exerc., 2001

[xxxix] Training Break "How quickly lose muscle", Mounir Azegra, 09/06/2021

Maintaining Physical Performance: The Minimal Dose of Exercise Needed to Preserve Endurance and Strength Over Time, Barry A Spiering, Iñigo Mujika, Marilyn A Sharp, Stephen A Foulis, J Strength Cond Res., 2021

[xl] Taking a complete break from resistance training for 2 weeks resulted no loss of muscle mass, Bill Campbell PhD, 26/12/2020 [xli] A biomechanical analysis of straight and hexagonal barbell Deadlifts using submaximal loads, Paul A Swinton, Arthur Stewart, Ioannis Agouris, Justin W L Keogh, Ray Lloyd, 2000-9,2011

Sci-sport : Soulevé de terre, une variante plus sûre pour tous les athlètes, P. Debraux, 2012

[xlii] La cellulite : comment l'irradier, voir, l'éradiquer ? TFK

Cellulite and its treatment, A V Rawlings, 2006

Cellulite: a review of its physiology and treatment, Mathew M Avram, 2004

[xliii] Squat Depth/variation do not affect glute activation, Strenght&Conditioning research, 2016

[xliv] Changes in rectus femoris architecture induced by the reverse Nordic hamstring exercices, Alonso-Fernandez & al., 2019 [xlv] Inhomogeneous architectural changes of the quadriceps femoris induced by resistance training, Ema & al., 2013

[xlvi] 3 mythes sur la fatigue du système nerveux central, Nevin, FitnessLogik (article web)

Fatigue : aspects psychophysiologiques, Les sites de la fatigue : périphériques et centraux, campusport. Univ-lille2 (article web) [xlvii] Acute neuromuscular and endocrine responses to two different compound exercises: squat versus deadlift, Barnes, Matthew J.; Miller, Adam; Reeve, Daniel; Stewart, Robin J.C.,2017 [xlviii] Comparison of upper body strength gains between men and women after 10 weeks of resistance training, PeerJ, 2016

[xlix] Comparison of hamstring and quadriceps femoris electromyographic activity between men and women during a singlelimb squat on both a stable and labile surface?, James W Youdas, John H Hollman, James R Hitchcock, Gregory J Hoyme, Jeremiah J

Johnsen, Journal of Strength and Conditioning Research 2007 [i] Être asymétrique est normal, Victor Depasse & Baptiste Gualiegue, 11 juin 2022, instagram

Les asymétries sont la norme, Remi Rvt, 5 juin 2022, instagram

Anatomic and functional leg-length inequality: A review and recommendation for clinical decision-making. Part I, anatomic leglength inequality: prevalence, magnitude, effects and clinical significance, Knutson, 2005

Comparing lumbo-pelvic kinematics in people with and without back pain: a systematic review and meta-analysis? Laird RA, 2014 Leg length discrepancy, Gurney B, 2002

[ii] Sex differences in resistance training : a systematic review and metaanalysis, Roberts, Nuckols & Krieger, 2020

Des résultats genrés : force & hypertrophie, M. Soulhol, instagram, 5 mai 2022

[iii] Déf. Athrose (médecine), Le Robert (dictonnaire)

[iiii] CHUV, service de neurochirurgie, « La douleur Chronique », site officiel

[liv] Delayed onset muscle soreness: treatment strategies and performance factors, Karoline Cheung, Patria Hume, Linda Maxwell, 2003

TFK, article 25 No pain no gain, Fausses idées Fitness & Nutrition [lv] Long Distance Running and Knee Osteoarthritis A Prospective Study, Eliza F. Chakravarty, Helen B. Hubert, Vijaya B. Lingala, Ernesto Zatarain,, and James F. Fries, 2008

[lvi] Running decreases knee intra-articular cytokine and cartilage oligomeric matrix concentrations: a pilot study (preview), Robert D. Hyldahl, Alyssa Evans, Sunku Kwon, Sarah T. Ridge, Eric Robinson, J. Ty Hopkins & Matthew K. Seeley, 2016 [lvii] Running exercise strengthens the intervertebral disc, Daniel L. Belavý, Matthew J. Quittner, Nicola Ridgers, Yuan Ling, David Connell & Timo Rantalainen, 2017

[lviii] TFK, art. 9 Tu ne perds pas de poids sur la balance, donc ton entraînement n'est pas efficace, Fausses idées Nutrition&Ftness

[lix] Cette mention est tirée de la recherche et de l'analyse d'article de « Health US News » ainsi que du e-book « Fausses idées Fitness&Nutrition », TFK

[lx] Effects of grip width on muscle strength and activation in the lat pull-down., Vidar Andersen, Marius S Fimland, Espen Wiik, Anders Skoglund, Atle H Saeterbakken 2014

La largeur de prise influence-t-elle le recrutement musculaire lors des tirages verticaux ? P. Debraux, 2014

[lxi] Pourquoi ça brûle ?, Marius Bzh, 29 avril 2020, IG

Unraveling the neurophysiology of muscle fatigue, Enoka & al, 2010

La fatigue périphérique : sites subcellulaires et mécanismes biologiques, J.D. Rouillon & R. Candau, em-consulte

[lxii] Aoi W, Marunaka Y. Importance of pH homeostasis in metabolic health and diseases: crucial role of membrane proton transport. Biomed Res Int. 2014

National Center for Biotechnology Information (2021). PubChem Compound Summary for CID 91435, Lactate. Modified June, 2022

L'acide lactique... ou pas ! Marius Bzh, 2021, IG

Nerdy muscle review "lactate innocent : deux décennies de lutte contre l'acidose métabolique, Remi Masson, pg 50-61, novembre 2019

[lxiii] Musculation et natation, Cometti, 2007

La pré-fatigue pour prendre du muscle, Marius Bzh, 29 juillet 2021, IG

[lxiv] La mind-muscle connection : Parce qu'il faut utiliser son cerveau en plus ?, Marius Bzh, 4 octobre 2021, IG

[lxv] Schoenfeld BJ, Vigotsky A, Contreras B, Golden S, Alto A, Larson R, Winkelman N, Paoli A. Differential effects of attentional focus strategies during long-term resistance training. Eur J Sport Sci. 2018 Jun;18(5):705-712.

[lxvi][lxvi] Wulf G. Attentional focus and motor learning: A review of 15 years. Int Rev Sport Exerc Psychol 6: 77–104, 2013.

[lxvii] Calatayud J, Vinstrup J, Jakobsen MD, Sundstrup E, Brandt M, Jay K, Colado JC, Andersen LL. Importance of mind-muscle connection during progressive resistance training. Eur J Appl Physiol. 2016 Mar;116(3):527-33.

[lxviii] Greig M, Marchant D. Speed dependant influence of attentional focusing instructions on force production and muscular activity during isokinetic elbow flexions. Hum Mov Sci. 2014 Feb;33:135-48.

[lxix] Effects of repetitions duration during resistance training on muscle hypertrophy : a systematic review on meta-analysis

[lxx] Fujita RA, Silva NRS, Bedo BLS, Santiago PRP, Gentil PRV, Gomes MM. Mind-Muscle Connection: Limited Effect of Verbal Instructions on Muscle Activity in a Seated Row Exercise. Percept Mot Skills. 2020 Oct;127(5):925-938

[lxxi] Baptiste Marchais : Big Back = big bench, Axel Ravinet, 2022, YT

Le recordman de développé couché me dévoile ses secrets pour soulever 230kg (ft. Bench&cigars), Nassim Sahili, 2022, YT [lxxii] Differences in the one-repetition maximum and load-velocity profile between the flat and arched bench press in competitive powerlifters, Sports Biomechanics, Garcia-Ramos & al., 2018 [lxxiii] Performance Differences Between the Arched and Flat Bench Press in Beginner and Experienced Paralympic Powerlifters, Neto & al, 2020

[lxxiv] Acute Effects of Posture Shirts on Rounded-Shoulder and Forward-Head Posture in College Students, John Manor, Elizabeth Hibberd, Meredith Petschauer, Joseph Myers, 2016

Effect of an exercise program for posture correction on musculoskeletal pain, DeokJu Kim, MiLim Cho, YunHee Park, and YeongAe Yang, 2015

The use of posture-correcting shirts for managing musculoskeletal pain is not supported by current evidence - a scoping review of the literature, Thorvaldur Skuli Palsson, Mervyn J Travers, Trine Rafn, Stian Ingemann-Molden, J P Caneiro, Steffan Wittrup Christensen, 2019

[lxxv] Subcutaneous Fat Alterations Resulting from an Upper-Body Resistance Training Program, Kostek & al. 2007

[lxxvi] Whole-body vibration exercise in postmenopausal osteoporosis, Magdalena Weber-Rajek,corresponding author Jan Mieszkowski, Bartłomiej Niespodziński, and Katarzyna Ciechanowska, 2015

Comparison of the Power Plate and Free Weight Exercises on Upper Body Muscular Endurance in College Age Subjects, Elisabeth Boland, Dan Boland, Thomas Carroll & William R. Barfield. Department of Health and Human Performance, College of Charleston, Charleston, SC, USA

Effects of 24 weeks of whole body vibration training on body composition and muscle strength in untrained females, M Roelants, C Delecluse, M Goris, S Verschueren, 2004

[lxxvii] Power Plate: Do Vibration Plates Work?, Exercise Biology : THE Science Of Exercise, 2010

[lxxviii] A comparitive study on stair walk and stepper strengthening exercise influence on the thigh muscle activation of university students, Kyung Mi Kim, Jin Seop Kim, Ji Heon Hong, Jae Ho Yu and Dong Yeop Lee, 2015

[lxxix] The effects of stepper exercise with visual feedback on strength, walking, and stair climbing in individuals following stroke, Munsang Choi, PT, MSc, Junsang Yoo, PT, MSc, Soonyoung Shin, JD and Wanhee Lee, 2015

[lxxx] "The effects of stepper exercise with visual feedback on strength, walking, and stair climbing in individuals following stroke", Munsang Choi, Junsang Yoo, Soonyoung Shin, Wanhee Lee, J Phys Ther Sci,2015 [lxxxi] L'éloge de la mastication, Hélène Baribeau, nutritionniste [lxxxii] The Relationship of Eating Rate and Degree of Chewing to Body Weight Status among Preschool Children in Japan: A Nationwide Cross-Sectional Study, Hitomi Okubo, Kentaro Murakami, Shizuko Masayasu, and Satoshi Sasaki, 2019

[lxxxiii] "Effects of Fat Grip Training on Muscular Strength and Driving Performance in Division I Male Golfers, Cummings, Patrick M.; Waldman, Hunter S.; Krings, Ben M.; Smith, John Eric W.; McAllister, Matthew J, 2018

[lxxxiv] Impact of Fat Grip Attachments on Muscular Strength and Neuromuscular Activation During Resistance Exercise, Krings & al., 2021

[lxxxv] Hypertension : L'isométrique au service de la santé cardiovasculaire, A. Manolova, 2022, Sci-sport

Smart NA, Way D, Carlson D, Millar P, McGowan C, Swaine I, Baross A, Howden R, Ritti-Dias R, Wiles J, Cornelissen V, Gordon B, Taylor R and Bleile B. Effects of isometric resistance training n resting blood pressure : Individual participant data meta-analysis. J Hypertens 37 : 1927-1938, 2019.

[lxxxvi] Grip Strength and Powerlifting Performance, Scot Morrison & al., 2010

[lxxxvii] Kinematic and EMG activities during front and back squat variations in maximum loads, Hasan Ulas Yavuz, Deniz Erdağ, Arif Mithat Amca & Serdar Aritan, Journal Of Sport Sciences, Pages 10581066, 2015

[lxxxix] A Biomechanical Comparison of Back and Front Squats in Healthy Trained Individuals, Gullett, Jonathan C; Tillman, Mark D; Gutierrez, Gregory M; Chow, John W, Journal of Strength and Conditioning Research, p 284-292, 2009

[xc] Electromyographic comparison of barbell deadlift, hex bar deadlift, and hip thrust exercises: a cross-over study, Andersen V, Fimland MS, Mo D-A, Iversen VM, Vederhus T, Rockland Hellebo LR, Nordaune KI and Saeterbakken AH., J Strength Cond Res, 587-593, 2018.

Comparaison de différents exercices pour l'activation des ischiojambiers et du grand fessier, A. Manolova, Sc-sport, 2018 [xci] Effects of a Six-Week Hip Thrust vs. Front Squat Resistance Training

Program on Performance in Adolescent Males: A Randomized Controlled Trial, Bret Contreras, Andrew D Vigotsky, Brad J Schoenfeld, Chris Beardsley, Daniel T McMaster, Jan H T Reyneke, John B Cronin, Journal of Strength and Conditioning Research, 999-1008, 2017

[xcii] Surface electromyographic activation patterns and elbow joint motion during a pull-up, chin-up, or perfect-pullupTM rotational exercise, Youdas JW, Amundson CL, Cicero KS, Hahn JJ, Harezlak DT and Hollman JH, J Strength Cond Res, 3404-3414, 2010

Différences de sollicitations musculaires entre tractions pronation et supination, P. Debraux, Sci-sport, 2014

[xciii] A comparative electromyographical investigation of muscle utilization patterns using various hand positions during the lat pulldown, Signorile JE, Zink AJ and Szwed SP, J Strength Cond Res, 539-546, 2002

[xciv] Biomechanical comparison of the reverse hyperextension machine and the hyperextension exercise, Michael A Lawrence, Andrew Chin, Brian T Swanson, J Strength Cond Res, 2053-2056, 2019.

[xcv] Comparaison biomécanique entre le Reverse Hyperextension et le Back Extension, P. Debraux, Sci-sport, 2019

[xcvi] Towards evidence based strength training: a comparison of muscle forces during deadlifts, goodmornings and split squats, Florian Schellenberg, William R. Taylor, and Silvio Lorenzetti, BMC Sports Sci Med Rehabil, 2017

[xcvii] Kinetic and kinematic differences between deadlifts and goodmornings, Florian Schellenberg, Julia Lindorfer, Renate List, William R Taylor & Silvio Lorenzetti, Sports Medicine, Arthroscopy, Rehabilitation, Therapy & Technology, art. 27, 2013.

[xcviii] Effects of body position and loading modality on muscle activity and strength in shoulder presses, Atle H Saeterbakken, Marius S Fimland, J Strength Cond Res, 1824-31, 2013 [xcix] Fausses idées Fitness&Nutrition, TFK, art. 30

[c] Blood Flow Restriction – The Holy Grail for Accessory Work?, Greg Nuckols, StrongerByScience, 2015 [ci] Blood Flow Restriction Resistance Training in Tendon Rehabilitation: A Scoping Review on Intervention Parameters, Physiological Effects, and Outcomes, Burton & al., Frontiers in Sports and Active Living, 2022

[cii] Effects of low-load resistance training with vascular occlusion on the mechanical properties of muscle and tendon, Keitaro Kubo& al., 112-9, 2006

[ciii] Effects of low load exercise with and without blood-flow restriction on microvascular oxygenation, muscle excitability and perceived pain, Kolind & al., J. of sport, 2022

[civ] Does blood flow restriction result in skeletal muscle damage? A critical review of available evidence, J. P. Loenneke R. S. Thiebaud T. Abe, Scandinavian Journal Of Medicine & Science In Sport, 2014 [cv] L'isométrie pour progresser en musculation, Christophe Collin, MyProtein, 2017

[cvi] Formation « Le système », Olivier Bolliet

[cvii] Xpertise 360 – formation Powerbuilding conjugué, Christian Thibaudeau

[cviii] ISOMETRICS FOR MASS! How to get bigger by not moving a muscle, Christian Thibaudeau, T. Nation, 2005

[cix] Kettlebell : Un peu de science dans un monde de fonte, P. Debraux & A. Manolova, Sci-sport, 2012

[cx] Elbow Extension Activation: Is there a difference with a pronated vs. supinated forearm?, answer of Leon Lategan, ResearchGate, 2016 [cxi] OVERHAND Vs UNDERHAND Tricep Extensions | What's Better?, Suneet Sebastian, Sebastian Fitness Solution

[cxii] Signorile JF, Zink AJ and Szwed SP. A Comparative Electromyographical Investigation of Muscle Utilization Patterns Using Various Hand Positions During the Lat Pull-down. J Strength Cond Res 16 (4) : 539-546, 2002.

Tirage nuque vs. tirage poitrine : quel est le plus efficace ?, P. Debraux,

Sci-sport, 2017

[cxiii] WHY ROTATING SHRUGS ARE CRAP, Christian Thibaudeau – Thibarmy, Youtube, 2019

[cxiv] Modifying a shrug exercise can facilitate the upward rotator muscles of the scapula, Pizzari T & al., Clin Biomech 29, 201-205, 2014

[cxv] Une variante de shrug pour mieux recruter ses trapèzes, P. Debraux, Sci-Sport, 2018

www.ingramcontent.com/pod-product-compliance
Lightning Source LLC
Chambersburg PA
CBHW071051240526
45471CB00015B/1558